BABY Friendly

MOTHER *Friendly*

EDITOR

Susan F. Murray

MA (Hons) Sociology, RN, RM

Lecturer in Maternal Health,
Centre for International Child Health,
Institute of Child Health, London

FOREWORD

Dr France Donnay

Women's Health Advisor, UNICEF, *New York*

ꟿ Mosby

London Baltimore Barcelona Bogotá Boston Buenos Aires Caracas Carlsbad, CA Chicago Madrid Mexico City Milan Naples, FL New York Philadelphia St. Louis Seoul Singapore Sydney Tai

618.2 MUR

Mosby titles of related interest:
Jones: *Ethics in Midwifery*, 1994
Richardson & Webber: *Ethical Issues in Child Health Care*, 1996
Dimond: *The Legal Aspects of Child Health Care*, 1996
Campbell & Glasper: *Whaley and Wong's Children's Nursing*, 1995

Project Manager:	Dave Burin
Cover Design/Designer:	Lara Last
Production:	Mike Heath
Layout Artist:	John Ormiston
Illustration:	Marion Tasker
Cover Illustration:	Deborah Gyan
Development Editor:	Hannah Tudge
Publisher:	Griselda Campbell

Published by Mosby, an imprint of Times Mirror International Publishers Limited

Printed in England by J W Arrowsmith Ltd

ISBN 0 7234 2123 4

For full details of all Times Mirror International Publishers Limited titles, please write to Times Mirror International Publishers Limited, Lynton House, 7–12 Tavistock Square, London WC1H 9LB, England.

A CIP catalogue record for this book is available from the British Library.

Contents

Contributors

Justina Nelago Amadhila is Senior Health Programme Administrator of the Nutrition Unit, Ministry of Health and Social Services, Namibia. She is a registered midwife with a BA in Nursing and a Diploma in Paediatric Nusing Science.

Sylvia Estrada-Claudio is a medical doctor and the co-coordinator of the Gabriela Commission on Women's Health and Reproductive Rights. Gabriela is a nationwide coalition of women's groups in the Philippines, comprising over 100 groups and 45,000 members.

G. Justus Hofmeyr is Professor and Head of the Department of Obstetrics and Gynaecology, Coronation Hospital and University of the Witwatersrand, Parktown, South Africa. He has a long-standing interest in 'woman-friendly' services, and he coordinated a randomized controlled trial of labour companions.

Saskia Kemp is a social anthropologist with a special interest in the social context of maternity care, has studied childhood issues and worked as a research assistant to Gabrielle Palmer.

Nicky Leap was formerly a community worker. She trained as a direct entry midwife in 1980 and since 1983 has worked as an independent midwife in London, specializing in home births. She is one of eight midwives who formed the South East London Midwifery Group Practice which became the first group practice to negotiate a contract with the National Health Service. She has produced two videos, *Helping You to Make Your Own Decisions*, antenatal and postnatal groups in Deptford, South East London, and *Home Birth Your Choice*. She has written extensively and is co-author of *Your Body, Your Baby, Your Life* (Pandora Press, 1983) and *The Midwife's Tale* (Scarlet Press, 1993).

Barbara Mensch is an Associate in the Research Division of the Population Council. A demographer, her most recent work has been in assessing the quality of care of reproductive health and family planning programmes in developing countries and in evaluating the impact of quality of care on reproductive behaviour. Prior to joining the Population Council, she was Assistant Professor of Clinical Public Health at Columbia University.

Maureen Minden is the MCH Coordinator for the American Refugee Committee Burmese Border Program in Thailand. She is a midwife, with a background in education and social anthropology. In the 1970s and 1980s she was involved in efforts to include midwifery as a profession in the Canadian health care system, a goal just now being realized. In 1986 she moved to the UK where she practised in the National Health Service. From 1989 to 1992 she was responsible for Mother and Child Health and for TBA training in the Kavre District of Nepal with Voluntary Service Overseas (VSO), and in 1993 she completed an MSc in Mother and Child Health at the Institute of Child Health, University of London. She is co-author of the English-language edition of Nepal's TBA training and supervision manual.

Ramona Alfaro Morales is a nurse midwife with many years of experience in the training of traditional midwives. She was an advisor on the Nicaraguan national TBA training manual. She is the Director of the Casa de Preparación para el Parto Natural in Estelí, and has been a prime advocate for active and natural birth techniques in Nicaragua.

Dikoloti Virginia Morewane is employed as a BFHI consultant by UNICEF. She also trains of health personnel in lactation management. In the past she has worked for the International Labour Organization on a programme for Improved Livelihood for Disabled Women. She has nursing and midwifery training and from 1984 to 1990 she was Supervisor and Senior Nursing Sister in charge of the Maternity Ward and MCH/FP Department of the National Referral and Training Hospital, Gaborone, Botswana.

Susan F. Murray is Lecturer in Maternal Health at the Centre for International Child Health, Institute of Child Health (University of London). She has training in midwifery, sociology and education. Her past experience includes hospital midwifery, administration of a mobile clinic, and coordination of a clinical trial, and from 1987 to 1990 she worked in Nicaragua in TBA training, active birth education, and education for reproductive health. She teaches and writes on Safe Motherhood issues and has travelled extensively. Her current research concerns the social construction of birth by caesarean section in Chile.

Suzanne Murray is a midwife with specialist training in breastfeeding support. She works at the Northpark Centre for Lactation Assessment, Resource and Education, Bundoora, Australia. She is author of *Breastfeeding Information and Guidelines*, a manual for breastmilk feeding support in paediatric and neonatal units (Royal Children's Hospital Parkville, Melbourne, 1992) and was a member of the State of Victoria Working Party for a Statewide Breastfeeding Protocol, published in 1994.

Daw Mya Mya is a Consultant to UNICEF and member of the BFHI Central Committee in Myanmar. She has been a member of the WHO expert advisory panel on Mother and Child Health since February 1993, is a member of the Overseas Reference Committee for the RCOG (UK), and was Head of the Institute of Medicine and Professor of Obstetrics and Gynaecology in Yangon, Myanmar until December 1988.

San San Myint is Consultant Paediatrician of the Special Care Baby Unit of the Central Women's Hospital in Yangon. She is also part time lecturer in Paediatrics at the Institute of Medicine. She is involved in the training of personnel for the BFHI and BFHD, and is a Wellstart Associate.

V. Cheryl Nikodem is Research Midwife and Lecturer in the Department of Obstetrics and Gynaecology, Coronation Hospital and University of the Witwatersrand, Parktown, South Africa.

Gabrielle Palmer is a specialist in breastfeeding. She is a policy advisor to Baby Milk Action (UK IBFAN) and is a member of the UK NGO Consortium on AIDS. She is author of *The Politics of Breastfeeding* (Pandora 1993), now in its second edition. She has worked in Mozambique, and has been a consultant for UNICEF, IBFAN, La Leche League and the Women's Environmental Network in many other countries. She runs a course in Breastfeeding Policy and Practice at the Institute of Child Health, University of London.

Patti Rundall is the international coordinator for Baby Milk Action, the UK member of IBFAN. She has worked on the protection of breastfeeding since 1980, playing an active role in the formation of European legislation and British law. She is a member of the UK government working party on infant feeding information. She is also the coordinator of the International Nestlé Boycott Committee and a trustee of the National Food Alliance.

Patricia Semeraro is a certified nurse-midwife currently working at the Rockville Centre, New York. She has been a midwife consultant to the Population Council for the last 8 years, working on various breastfeeding and post-partum projects. She is a co-author of the Population Council publication, *Contraception during breastfeeding: A Clinician's Sourcebook.*

Diana G. Smith BSc(Econ), is editor of *Contact*, the health journal of the World Council of Churches, Geneva, and former editor of the *Safe Motherhood Newsletter* of the World Health Organization. She visited the Gabriela project in Apelo Cruz in October 1992.

Penny Van Esterik is an anthropologist, teaching at York University, Canada. She is the author of *Motherpower and Infant Feeding* (Zed Press), *Women, Work and Breasfeeding* (Cornell International Nutrition Monographs), and other work on gender and food. She is the coordinator of the Task Force on Breastfeeding and Women's Work for WABA (World Alliance for Breastfeeding Action).

Esther H. Viljoen is qualified in general nursing and midwifery. She was one of Namibia's Internal Assessors for evaluating progress made in promoting breastfeeding in the country. She is also a director in Johanniter Health Work (a non-governmental organization), preparing a module for Home Care Workers.

Foreword

There is very good news in this interesting and informative book. Readers will first learn a great deal about one of the most serious threats to young child survival and normal development: our increasingly slippery grasp on breastfeeding, the anchor of infant feeding, health, and care. Before despair takes hold, however, relief comes in the form of solutions as evident and pervasive as the problem. We are reassured here, through professional accounts more reminiscent of personal testimonies than programme reports, that humankind has lost neither the skill of breastfeeding nor the age-old knowledge of how best to assist women through childbirth, the everyday event that is nonetheless phenomenal. We have just temporarily lost sight of their value and misplaced them among the trappings of medicalisation. This excellent text offers willing travellers a road map back to the point where common sense and respect for nature prevail over our fascination with medicine.

UNICEF views reproductive health and women's issues as indivisible from child survival, health, and development. Breastfeeding is a bridge between the woman and child, and the importance of that bridge to our very survival, and the role of health workers in keeping the bridge intact and weightbearing, warrant the careful attention given by this book, and more.

Nature ensures that when a woman gives birth, she develops the inherent capacity to provide her child with food, health protection, and care. But today, beginning moments after childbirth and even sooner, access to that natural resource is made difficult or impossible for many women by a number of obstacles - every one of which is man-made. A new mother may face cultural and family pressure not to breastfeed; she may find herself forced to choose between her baby's welfare and her own when political decisions limit her maternity leave; and she will almost certainly be subjected to modern myths, such as 'the insufficient milk syndrome', that will cast a shadow over her confidence and question her competence. Full informatioon about the benefits of breastfeeding, the risks of not breastfeeding, and the dangers of using infant formula may be withheld from her, or the facts may be distorted by ignorance or intentional manipulation. The more industrialized her society, the more likely a woman may be able to find that modern knowledge and state-of-the-art practices exist elsewhere in her health system, but that maternity care practices are outdated, management of the birth process is invasive, and maternity care providers are misinformed.

Baby Friendly Hospitals, models of modern maternity care in settings around the world, create environments that restore to women their authority over breastfeeding, their own natural resource. Newcomers to the iniative will find several historic 'firsts' in the WHO/UNICEF Baby Friendly Hospital Initiative (BFHI) - including its distinction as the first global nutrition programme to place *beneficiaries* in charge. BFHI's design ensures that only if and when *mothers* have determined, through their personal experience, that a hospital's maternity care practices have satisfactorily met the established criteria for designation can a hospital receive the distinguished BFHI global award.

BFHI has also played the role of maverick by opening up health systems to the scrutiny and judgement of their users. In a participatory way that is unusual in today's health institutions, mothers, midwives, and other central players in the age-old rituals of childbirth have found in the BFHI a window onto the tightly controlled and closed domain of national health systems.

Readers in search of a recipe for empowerment will recognize its ingredients in the Baby Friendly Hospital Initiative, as seen through the eyes of midwives and described so vividly in this book: access to facts and information, the right to informed choice and real options from which to choose.

Dr France Donnay
Women's Health Advisor, UNICEF, New York

Preface

These are exciting and thought-provoking times. Midwifery internationally is in a state of flux. New developments affecting midwifery practice and research in developing and industrialized countries, have brought with them challenge and conflict. There are tensions between lay women's knowledge and power and medicalization, between traditional caring functions and professionalization, between individual care perspectives and public health perspectives, and between the need to provide services that are accessible and acceptable and the harsh economic realities of today's world. These themes run through many of the contributions to these two companion volumes, and the perspectives offered are rich and varied. Some chapters give an international overview of particular themes and are written by experts in those particular fields; others are written by experienced midwives and nurse-midwives who give concrete examples of the phenomena in question in a particular real life setting.

In the choice of contributors and themes, I used as starting points the two major global initiatives that have most impacted on international midwifery practice in recent years, the Safe Motherhood Initiative and the Baby Friendly Hospital Initiative. With the edited contributions I have tried to bring together the theory and the practice of midwifery. I refer to these in their broadest sense: not only theoretical concepts in midwifery but theory about midwifery; not only clinical midwifery practice but the practice of midwifery policy and midwifery research. The books were written in the main by midwives themselves with their own profession in mind, but they also recognize the contribution that other disciplines, particularly the social sciences, can make to our understanding of what and who we are.

Much of the material in these volumes highlights the ways in which women across the world still lack power in relation to their own bodies, their own fertility and their own babies. Some of this powerlessness is the product of wider societal forces, of economic systems, of traditional beliefs, of modern commercial interests. Some of the responsibility, as many of the authors point out very clearly, also has to be laid directly at the door of the Western medical system and its advocates and implementers. Midwives must accept that we too have played our part in this. Our challenge now, as we approach the millennium, is to thoughtfully reconsider our role in the care of the health of women and their babies, and with this our role as women's advocates. Midwives have the potential of a unique and privileged relationship with women during important life events. This is something to be treasured. However, to my mind it is increasingly clear that we cannot confine our horizons to the provision of good individual care alone. Unique and privileged relationships bring with them wider social responsibilities and functions, to document, to research, to debate, to defend, and to advocate.

Susan F. Murray

Introduction

'Quality of care' is a much-debated and contested term. Maxwell suggested the following aspects to quality of care: access to services, relevance to need for the whole community, equity, social acceptability, effectiveness, efficiency, and economy [Maxwell, R.J. (1994) Quality assessment in health. *British Medical Journal*, **288**: 1470–1471]. However in many parts of the world, particularly in under-resourced maternity services, the term is still used to refer to little more than technical practices, and other issues such as patient–provider interaction are not considered to be so important (see Chapter 13). This narrow perspective is being challenged, in various creative ways. The contributions to this edited volume invite the reader to consider application of 'quality of care' to midwifery in practice, through overviews of certain thematic issues and through specific case studies from across the world.

The first section of the volume (Chapters 1–7) takes as its starting point one of the major global initiatives to have affected midwifery in recent years, the Baby Friendly Hospital Initiative (BFHI). This was launched by the United Nations Children's Fund (UNICEF) in 1991 in a campaign to motivate all health facilities to implement the 'Ten Steps to Successful Breastfeeding' (see Chapter 1, Appendix II). The Initiative focused on what happened in hospitals after birth because this was where many of the barriers to breastfeeding promotion occurred. It incorporated in its design a notion of quality of midwifery care that is both technical and relational, with its emphasis on the protection, promotion, and support of breastfeeding.

The first part of the book concerns the ways in which this concept of 'baby friendliness' can be achieved in practice. In Chapter 1, Gabrielle Palmer and Saskia Kemp give an outline of the history of the medicalization of infant feeding, and make a strong argument for the need for breastfeeding promotion and for the BFHI. They then go on to raise very important questions as to the role of the professional midwife within this. As more research is carried out in order to inform breastfeeding policy and practice, the issue of who is seen as 'the expert' is a particularly challenging one. A fine balance has to be maintained between the need to be a well-informed professional and the need to preserve power in the hands in which it belongs – those of the breastfeeding mother. The theme of midwife as enabler or disempowerer is revisited later in the book by Nicky Leap (Chapter 12).

Chapters 2–5 provide us with case studies from different countries, developed and developing, to illustrate the practical application of the BFHI 'on the ground', and which show how the model of 'Ten Steps to Successful Breastfeeding' can be modified to suit individual country or community circumstances. Dikoloti Morewane starts with an example from Botswana of a highly successful 'baby friendly' initiative in a maternity unit which long predated the global UNICEF campaign. Suzanne Murray describes the situation in Australia, one quite typical for an industrialized and wealthy country, and demonstrates how the 'Ten Steps' were introduced in a private hospital there. Daw Mya Mya and San San Myint explain why, with UNICEF, they developed a Baby Friendly Home Delivery Initiative project in Myanmar (previously known as Burma). Finally, Esther Viljoen and Justina Amadhila outline Namibia's National Baby *and Mother* Friendly Initiative.

Sometimes, particularly in the West, it is argued that infant feeding is just a matter of personal choice. Patti Rundall gives us a graphic description in Chapter 6 of the reasons why such an approach is too simplistic, and why breastfeeding needs to be protected (as well as promoted and supported), in her account of the commercial pressures against breastfeeding.

Midwives, of course, are often mothers too! This is something seldom considered, even by those progressive health-service managers who wish their staff to promote breastfeeding in their professional capacity. Many midwives encounter little opportunity to breastfeed their own children successfully on returning to work. In Chapter 7, Penny Van Esterik takes up this issue, and gives some ideas and examples from different countries of how this situation can be tackled.

One of the limitations of high-impact, focused campaigns, such as the BFHI, is what, or who, they leave out. Some countries, like Namibia as discussed in Chapter 5, have begun to take on board the fact that 'mother friendliness' – the provision of facilities and services that are acceptable and accessible to women – is the corollary to any successful breastfeeding initiative. Women also need to feel happy and confident in using the available maternity and reproductive health services, if safer motherhood (the reduction of maternal mortality and morbidity) is to be achieved. The second half of this volume takes up this theme, and examines some of the different ways in which 'mother friendliness' may be achieved.

Chapters 8–10 consider ways in which the quality of maternity services can be measured from the point of view of acceptability to women users. Many maternity units across the world still refuse women the right to have someone to accompany them throughout their labour and delivery. Justus Hofmeyr and Cheryl Nikodem (Chapter 8) provide an excellent review of the evidence from randomized trials that having a labour companion can improve the labour outcome. They then describe the controlled trial that they themselves conducted in South Africa, which demonstrated the positive impact that having a companion in labour can have on successful and confident breastfeeding.

Many developing-country hospitals have limited resources and an extremely high turnover of patients. This does make personalized care more difficult, but not necessarily as impossible as some would have us believe. Maureen Minden (Chapter 9) gives a very frank and disturbing description of the situation for women using a maternity hospital in Nepal, which receives 15,000 obstetric admissions per year, and makes some clear suggestions of how the needs of these women could be better met.

Sometimes ideas seem so entrenched and obstacles so huge that even the well-intentioned midwife feels that there is little hope of changing anything. Ramona Alfaro Morales's chapter defies any such pessimism. She describes the evolution of a small- scale project run by nurses and midwives in northern Nicaragua, which set out to improve both the physical and the emotional care given to women by the health services and by traditional midwives. That many of these developments took place during a period of great instability, economic blockade and guerilla warfare make the project all the more inspiring.

When health services are poor and disrespectful, some women learn to keep their heads down and accept the indignities with a degree of resignation. Many others vote with their feet. They either do not attend at all, or they use services only in emergencies. Other women get organized! In Chapter 11, Diana Smith and Sylvia Estrada-Claudio give us a fascinating account of how a women's organization in the Philippines took action when state health services failed to meet the needs of poor women from the shanty town. The Gabriela Women's Health Commission has gone on to develop a new vision of appropriate health services for women.

Chapter 12 also takes up this theme of appropriate maternity care, but in the context of a highly technologized and well-resourced Western health system. Nicky Leap gives a vivid account of the changing face of the maternity services in Britain, and of the first midwifery group practice to win a health authority contract. She makes an impassioned argument for the potential of woman-led midwifery care, and for the role of the midwife in enabling and empowering "through doing as little as possible".

The final chapter, by Patricia Semeraro and Barbara Mensch, addresses the underlying theme of this volume, and looks at how quality of care might be defined for antenatal and reproductive health services. They describe the framework that the Population Council is currently field-testing for use in the assessment of such services, and they suggest how this can then be used by midwives to improve care provision.

Acknowledgements

I wish to express my warm thanks to the many people who contributed to the two volumes of International Perspectives on Midwifery. Much labour went into these pages, and I know that for many of the authors this was done a little wearily, at the end of long working days, or nights, full of other priorities and commitments, and at the mercy of erratic power supplies and unreliable postal services.

I would particularly like to thank Helen Armstrong, Gabrielle Palmer, Barbara Kwast, and Joan Walker for their invaluable initial suggestions on contributors. I also wish to thank Fiona Watson whose incisive assistance in editing at a crucial moment helped to save the books from foundering, and Della R. Sherratt, Head of Overseas Education Developments, Avon and Gloucester College of Health, whose comments as the publisher's referee were immensely valuable.

Dedication

To the memory of Ann Garner, who I will always think of as 'my' midwife, and who knew all about leading "so that the mother is still free and in charge".

CHAPTER

1

Breastfeeding Promotion and the Role of the Professional Midwife

Gabrielle Palmer and **Saskia Kemp**

> *... I have given suck, and know*
> *How tender 'tis to love the babe that milks me*
> *(William Shakespeare, Lady Macbeth, Act 1, Scene 7)*

INTRODUCTION

We would not need to promote breastfeeding if so much were not happening to impede it. If we look at non-human mammals, no mother fails to suckle her young *unless something drastic has occurred to impede the natural progress of birth and rearing.* It is striking that primates in zoos who have not been mothered themselves and have never experienced or witnessed breastfeeding are unable to care for their own infants; this ineptness is passed on to the next generation (Elia, 1985). We have to ask whether something similar has happened to humans in those societies where mothering skills, such as breastfeeding, no longer seem spontaneous.

Breastfeeding spans both the arenas of eating and drinking and of sexual activity (in the sense of physical pleasure and sensuality); also, in common with other areas to do with food and sex, it has been subject to social control and interference. A common knowledge about breastfeeding existed until relatively recently. William Shakespeare, the famous English playwright, knew that women enjoyed breastfeeding and that the baby was the active stimulator of the milk, because in his time (late sixteenth, early seventeenth century) it was common knowledge. That knowledge has been lost.

We have to promote breastfeeding because human society has damaged it. Promotion therefore involves acting to prevent certain activities more than it does preaching and pushing. Take away the constraints that impede breastfeeding and there would be no need to promote it. This was acknowledged in *The Innocenti Declaration* (1990) – see Appendix I, pages 17–18 – a summary of investigations made during the 1980s by six specialist working groups sponsored by international agencies:

> *Efforts should be made to increase women's confidence in their ability to breastfeed.*
> *Such empowerment involves the removal of constraints and influences that*

manipulate perceptions and behaviour towards breastfeeding, often by subtle and indirect means. This requires sensitivity, continued vigilance, and a responsive and comprehensive communications strategy involving all media and addressed to all levels of society. Furthermore, obstacles to breastfeeding within the health system, the workplace, and the community must be eliminated.

Breastfeeding is an emotional subject; it touches the core of all of us because our early feeding was our primary experience of a relationship. It is a biological inheritance, yet is profoundly influenced by social and economic structures. The medicalization of such a sensitive personal experience has damaged this vital human activity and the commercial exploitation of medical misunderstanding has entrenched this damage. How can the midwife promote breastfeeding in a world where powerful forces beyond her control work against it?

WHY PROMOTE BREASTFEEDING?

Research in the past two decades has revealed increasing advantages for breastfeeding, both for mothers and babies. Many midwives know that tired phrase, 'breast is best', but defending this claim with scientific evidence can be hard. The fact that we find ourselves in a world where we have to prove the real thing is better than the substitute illustrates the craziness of the situation that we face. It is useful to touch upon just a few of the reasons why breastfeeding is worth promoting.

Recent reviews of the scientific literature show that breastfeeding can save more lives and prevent more morbidity than any other health strategy (Lutter, 1990). Breast milk contains an ideal balance of nutrients for complete body and brain growth, but it is more than a food; it is a multi-purpose medicine, rich in anti-infection factors which protect the baby against disease (for a detailed account of the biochemistry and immunological significance of human milk, see Lawrence, 1994). Breastfed babies are less likely to suffer from infections than babies fed breastmilk substitutes. It is not merely a matter of hygiene; even in the best conditions, a baby who is not breastfed is five times more likely to suffer gastro-intestinal illness (Howie *et al.*, 1990). In difficult conditions, where diarrhoeal diseases are commonplace, a bottle-fed child is 14 times more likely to die than a breastfed one. There is a dose-related risk to this mortality, the mixed fed child having a higher risk the lower the proportion of breastfeeding to artificial feeding (Victora *et al.*, 1989).

Exclusive breastfeeding in the first 4–6 months is important, because any other fluid, food, or even a dummy can interfere with the process, both through the risk of infection and by reducing the baby's suckling. Early initiation, breastfeeding on demand, and breastfeeding exclusively are all important to establish lactation. Continued breast-milk production is controlled by the baby; the more effectively he or she suckles, the more milk is made. Breast milk adapts to the climate so that the proportion of fluid meets the baby's needs in relation to temperature and humidity (WHO Working Group on Infant Feeding, 1991). Water, or any other fluid, is not only unnecessary, but is a risk for the baby (WHO Working Group on Infant Feeding, 1992a). After 6 months the baby needs solid food too, but breastfeeding for 2 years and beyond ensures both a balanced diet and disease protection and, in many parts of the world, survival (Briend *et al.*, 1988).

Exclusively breastfed babies can become ill, but disease severity is less than in artificially fed babies. During outbreaks of diarrhoea and acute respiratory infection, it is mostly those who are not breastfed who have to be hospitalized (Fallot *et al.*, 1980). Breastfeeding reduces the risk of a wide range of conditions, including urinary tract infections (Piscane *et al.*, 1990), ear infections (Facione, 1990), early onset diabetes (Mayer *et al.*, 1988), allergy (Merrett *et al.*, 1988), and sudden infant death syndrome (SIDS or cot death; Mitchell *et al.*, 1991). Breastfed children score better in mental development tests right through to school age (Rogan and Gladen, 1993). For premature babies, deaths from necrotizing enterocolitis are reduced significantly (Lucas and Cole, 1990). A breastfed child's body makes better use of immunization (Hahn-Zoric *et al.*, 1990), and she or he is less likely to suffer childhood cancer (Davis *et al.*, 1988) or bowel disease (Koletzko *et al.*, 1989). Though later diet and life-style are important too, breastfeeding may protect against coronary heart disease (Barker and Osmond, 1986) and teeth will be better formed (Labbock and Hendershot, 1987).

Breastfeeding helps protect women's health: in the short-term, the uterus returns to its pre-pregnancy size and there may be hormonal benefits – for example, when a diabetic woman breastfeeds, she needs less insulin. In the long-term, the risk of breast and ovarian cancer can be reduced (Brock *et al.*, 1989; Davies *et al.*, 1989; UK National Case-Control Study Group, 1993). Breastfeeding inhibits ovulation. As long as a woman breastfeeds frequently and exclusively, and as long as she has no menstruation, in the first 6 months after childbirth there is a 98% protection from pregnancy, which is equivalent to other modern methods of child spacing (WHO Working Group on Infant Feeding, 1992b).

Skin contact stimulates the hormones, which can trigger maternal feelings (Karolinska Institute, 1991). There are many ways in which parents and babies 'fall in love' with each other, but the cuddling and closeness of breastfeeding seems to enhance these feelings. In some countries where breastfeeding has improved due to changed hospital practices, there has been a reduction in the abandonment of babies (UNICEF, 1992).

Breastfeeding brings economic and environmental benefits. For many people, to feed a baby with commercial baby milk would cost almost an entire salary. For example, in Kenya the cost of purchasing commercial breast-milk substitutes, not including the bottles, fuel, and water would require 91% of an agricultural worker's wage (Savage King, 1992). In the United States, the government spends at least US$30 million a year on artificial milk for low-income mothers, providing 40% of the baby food industry's US market (Riordan and Auerbach, 1993). In France, the cost of extra hospital admissions due to artificial feeding has been conservatively estimated to be over 71 million francs (about US$12 million; Bitoun, 1994). Over a decade ago it was calculated that if 25% of Indonesian women stopped breastfeeding, an extra $40 million would have to be spent on diarrhoeal treatment and an extra $80 million on family planning services. The importation of baby feeding products wastes scarce foreign exchange in developing countries. Packaging, bottles, teats, and the fuel for sterilization all create unnecessary pollution and waste when the superior product is available in women's breasts (Rohde, 1982; Radford, 1992).

The common belief that many women cannot produce enough milk is mistaken. All women are equipped to feed twins. Indeed, triplets and even quadruplets have been fully breastfed (Carson, 1992). The majority of women who thought they could not breastfeed did not have a physiological malfunction, which is rare, but suffered from misinformation and a lack of emotional support. Maternal diet is not crucial to breastfeeding in the way that it is to healthy pregnancy (Prentice *et al.*, 1986). Scientists have discovered that human lactation is a resilient process, withstanding adverse conditions so long as the baby suckles frequently and effectively. In disaster situations, infants often survive better than older children because of breastfeeding (Kelly, 1993).

THE MEDICALIZATION OF INFANT FEEDING

It is with great Pleasure I see at last the Preservation of Children become the Care of Men of Sense. In my opinion, this Business has been too long fatally left to the management of Women, who cannot be supposed to have a proper Knowledge to fit them for the Task, notwithstanding they look upon it to be their own Province. (William Cadogan, 1748)

William Cadogan, called 'the father of paediatrics', was an influential doctor whose writings were reprinted and translated throughout Europe. By 'men of sense' William Cadogan meant doctors like himself. Women had little access to education at this time, but they carried a store of undocumented knowledge, particularly about child care, which, as Cadogan grumblingly acknowledged, they considered 'their own Province'. Cadogan and his followers did not suggest improving women's education, and for the next 200 years male medical doctors became increasingly influential in the field of infant feeding.

This culture of scorn for women's child-rearing skills persisted into the twentieth century. Another influential doctor, Sir Frederick Truby King, was an advocate of breastfeeding but a promoter of rigid routines and restricted physical contact. He argued (King, 1913):

Were the secretion of milk and the feeding of the baby the functions of men and not women, no man – inside or outside the medical profession – would nurse his baby more than five times in the twenty four hours ...

Despite this claimed superiority, these doctors never felt compelled to take on baby care. To this day in all societies baby care is still undertaken principally by women, whether they are mothers, grandmothers, and aunts or health professionals, nursery staff, and child minders. Artificial feeding, which could be viewed as the means of enabling men to take complete care of babies, is still predominantly carried out by women, either the mother or a substitute carer. The baby's welfare has been and is still viewed as the mother's responsibility, even if she delegates that responsibility. In the past a mother substitute would have also breastfed the baby (wet nursing). In most of the world baby care is a low-status job, both in terms of pay and prestige.

From Cadogan's time, medical men (the few women doctors dared not challenge medical orthodoxy and risk losing the grudging recognition they had struggled so hard to gain) have influenced the 'rules of management' of breastfeeding, for better or for worse. Cadogan noted that the breastfed babies of working-class English women thrived. In contrast, the babies of the rich received pre-lacteal feeds of butter and honey, sugared wine, or water (Fildes, 1986) and then were sent to a wet nurse, or even artificially fed, with inevitably tragic results. Pre-lacteal feeds, whether local products or commercial dextrose or glucose water, have been (and are still) used in both traditional and industrialized societies (Morse *et al.*, 1990). It seems there is a strong impulse to intervene with new babies (Elia, 1985).

One reason for this avoidance of maternal breastfeeding by aristocratic women was the awareness of the negative effect of breastfeeding on fertility. They had to produce many heirs and had less control over their bodies than poorer women who consciously used breastfeeding of both their own and other babies as a means of fertility control (Palmer, 1993). Cadogan educated the English upper classes about the life-saving effect of early exclusive breastfeeding and the risks of pre-lacteal feeds; both infant and maternal mortality fell as a result. Avoidance of pre-lacteal feeds leads to a lowering of early infection rates. The fall in maternal mortality could be explained by improved expulsion of the placenta, reduction in postpartum bleeding, and less engorgement and consequent mastitis, which could have led to septicaemia and death.

Despite his observational skills, Cadogan made mistakes. He decided that 'overfeeding' caused infant diarrhoea (the germ theory of disease was not discovered until the nineteenth century) and he did not distinguish between breast milk and other foods when he promoted his theory. He advocated only four feeds at regular intervals during the 24 hours and forbade night feeding. Fortunately, he did not suggest limiting the duration of a feed. Until the mid-eighteenth century, no one had considered restricting a baby's access to the breast. Such is Cadogan's influence that his one disastrous idea, that of restricting feeding episodes, is still attempted wherever Western medical influence has superseded cultural norms.

For the 200 years following Cadogan, as the medical profession became more powerful and as childbirth and the postnatal period came to be supervised by doctors and systems of health surveillance, so the arbitrary whim of one man became a rule and eventually accepted custom. Ironically, the very edict imposed to prevent overfeeding caused underfeeding; only a few lucky babies could stimulate sufficient milk under these restrictions. The mothers who obeyed medical advice by restricting the number of feeds found that their milk decreased and were grateful when the doctors suggested supplements based on cows' milk. They also became dependent on doctors to guide them through the hazards of artificial feeding. Many babies died as a result of not being breastfed but, as conditions improved, more survived the risks. Consequently, the practice became more acceptable. Doctors could test out theories concerning artificial feeding on babies of the richer women who believed they could not breastfeed. Poor women could not afford doctors nor the conditions for preparing the risky artificial foods, so their babies died in greater numbers. Thus, despite economic growth, more food, fuel, and medical knowledge, infant mortality rates in Europe and North America increased during the final decades of the nineteenth century (Palmer, 1993).

By the 1920s the health professions were intimately connected with the use of commercial breast-milk substitutes. A relationship evolved between the milk manufacturers and doctors. One example among many is that of the British Paediatric

Association (BPA), which has accepted funding from baby food companies since the 1920s. Many midwives' and nurses' professional bodies have also become dependent on such sponsorship. It has become normal for health professionals to accept such funding, making it that bit harder for the professional to speak out when a company's practices are unethical. This relationship, described by the late D. Derrick Jelliffe as "Endorsement by association, manipulation by assistance," has clouded infant feeding policies all over the world (Jeliffe and Jeliffe, 1978). As the twentieth century progressed a benign acceptance of the inevitability of artificial feeding became established.

Some doctors were pro-breastfeeding, but their misunderstanding of the way women's bodies worked made many of them inept at dealing with any breastfeeding difficulty. It seemed that each new medical rule sabotaged the process. These rules included separation of mother and baby in hospital, curtailment of the frequency *and duration* of breastfeeds, the washing of nipples, and the giving of pre-lacteal and supplementary artificial feeds. Cadogan's good concepts were abandoned, but his harmful ones became entrenched. It is now known that the restriction of the frequency of feeds shuts down milk production and that the restriction of the duration of a feed impedes the baby's access to the important hind milk. Similarly, it is now clear that sore nipples are not caused by prolonged or frequent feeding, but by incorrect attachment of the baby at the breast, by excessive washing of the nipples, and sometimes by *Candida albicans* infection. Because of the influence of bottle-feeding, both health professionals and mothers came to position babies as though for bottle-feeding and offer the nipple as though it were an artificial teat. As early as 1903, a leading US paediatrician, Dr Koplick, showed his ignorance of the physiology of human lactation (Koplick, 1903):

> *The thumb may be used to exert pressure on the breast, thus aiding the flow of milk. In this way the infant is prevented from drawing the nipple too far into the mouth.*

Influenced by such health professionals and their followers, women lost their skill in helping the baby to take a good mouthful at the breast.

As public breastfeeding (and visible breastfeeding within the household) disappeared, the subliminal education of observation was denied and the unconscious skills and knowledge died. Having been breastfed by one's own mother influences breastfeeding practice. The package of rules established with medicalized childbirth, when combined with the demise of social and emotional support, led to the artificial-feeding societies we find today. The huge financial profits available from marketing breast-milk substitutes have established a vested interest in maintaining this lamentable situation.

These rules were invented by men, whose lack of personal experience makes their mistakes understandable. The rules were implemented by women health professionals (nurses and midwives), who deferentially accepted that male doctors knew more than women who had breastfed. As the power of doctors increased, midwives became increasingly scorned. In the United States and Canada they were outlawed and, although this situation is changing, their influence today is still marginalized by the medical establishment. In most of Europe, midwives were saved by becoming professionals themselves (e.g., Public and General Act (1902), Midwives Act), which involved some sacrifice of autonomy and an absorption into the hegemony of medicine and nursing.

Doctors told mothers how to feed their babies either directly or indirectly through midwives and nurses. Mothers were expected to obey and the fear of infant death assisted this compliance. There is no doubt that the twentieth century improvement in industrialized nations' living conditions, health services, and education helped save infants' and children's lives, but harm accompanied the good. Hospitalized childbirth was not the blessing it was made out to be and in the United States birth injuries increased with hospital births (Oakley, 1984). The regimes, nurseries, and bottles that accompanied hospital childbirth almost destroyed breastfeeding. Women's faith in and reverence for doctors prevented them from discerning the harm.

In the UK in 1896 the Health Visitors' Association was established to carry health messages to 'ignorant' mothers. Some useful knowledge was spread, but a culture was established whereby it was assumed that mothers could not rear their children without the guidance of experts. The effect on breastfeeding was negative, not for lack of enthusiasm for its superiority over artificial feeding, but because health visitors dutifully promoted the doctors' rules. Mothers were told that their ways were wrong. In a 1907 report, a health visitor described the success of her persuasions: "Why," said one woman who at last understood the meaning of regular feeding, "I have had five children and no one has ever told me that before" (Barnett, 1907). Women in remoter areas escaped the health visitors, but were regarded as ignorant, as this woman who had brought up her children during the World War I (1914–1918) and after, "We didn't have no bottle for our children. Fed them all ourselves. Every one. All nine. Till they were 3 years old some of them. ... I didn't know, see" (Chamberlain, 1983).

The misguided health education spread around the world through colonialism. In Malaysia in 1926 British nurses reported that, "some mothers had not even seen a clock and those who had could not understand what it had to do with the feeding of an infant" (King and Ashworth, 1987a). In the Caribbean in 1917, British Colonial Nurses complained about women breastfeeding into the second year, "No amount of advice will prevent them from carrying on this deadly habit" (King and Ashworth, 1987b). Without scientific evidence, doctors had decided that breast milk contained no nutritive value after 1 year and strongly discouraged continued breastfeeding. The United States introduced their medical model of childbirth and made bottle-feeding routine in the Philippines and Latin America. Wherever Western health practices were introduced, breastfeeding suffered and the baby food and bottle companies followed in their wake.

THE LEGACY OF MEDICALIZATION

Since breastfeeding had been made difficult many women did 'fail' to breastfeed. This led to a mass loss of confidence in women's bodies, which in turn influenced individual women to doubt their own power. They turned to the 'supplementary' bottle, and when their breast milk inevitably lessened, they blamed their own bodies. This widespread belief in mammary impotence is a tragedy, not just for the babies, but for the women who have endured the sense of failure.

There have been some efforts to change the harmful practices over the years. In 1942, a British Government Report (Ministry of Health, 1942) stated that the establishment of breastfeeding was less successful in hospital than after home birth. The report noted that babies were weighed too frequently, given supplementary bottles too readily, and that routines were too rigid. Modern research has vindicated these recommendations (RCM, 1991; WHO, 1993), but such is the resistance to change that the global strategy of UNICEF's Baby Friendly Hospital Initiative (BFHI) with *The Ten Steps to Successful Breastfeeding* (WHO/UNICEF, 1989); see Appendix II, page 19) has had to be launched to implement changes that have been known to be important for more than 50 years. Despite the thoroughness which went into the formulation of *The Ten Steps*, which are based on the research available at the time, implementation has been slow, especially in industrialized countries.

"The fact that a practice cannot be shown to be of benefit ought to be sufficient reason for abandoning it, especially in the present economic climate" (RCM, 1991), yet implementors of the BFHI say that changing the practices of health professionals can be harder than convincing mothers of the benefits of breastfeeding. It is remarkable how fiercely medical systems cling to old rituals with no scientific justification. If we consider the changes in surgical techniques, from dirty knife to laser beam, over the past 100 years, it is astonishing that we are still sustaining practices established through the random fancies of long-dead doctors. For example, supplementary and complementary feeds, of either water, glucose and/or dextrose, or formula have not been shown in any randomized controlled trials to be of benefit to healthy, breastfed infants (RCM, 1991). Yet many doctors, midwives, and nurses are more fearful of allowing a baby free access to the breast than of performing the unjustified ritual of giving a bottle of fluid. We must ask why the health establishment suffers from such irrational conservatism in this area.

These medical mistakes could not have endured if the marketing practices of the commercial baby food and bottle companies had not exploited them. Women whose breastfeeding establishment had been undermined in the hospital, their confidence shaken, went home and fell prey to promotion, often initiated in the hospital. Thousands of health workers have helped the baby food and bottle companies increase their sales by offering mothers artificial feeds and by giving them milk and equipment to take home. It is now clear that the likelihood of milk insufficiency is extremely rare so long as the suckling technique is correct. In the case of babies unable to suckle, mothers can maintain sufficient breast milk if they are given good practical help with the techniques of milk expression and emotional support.

Those who have educated themselves through intelligent observation or available materials may be forced to continue with these impeding practices because of the power of the medical establishment or commercial political forces. For example, in Canada, at the Women's Hospital in Toronto, health professionals tried to resist a hospital contract whereby Mead Johnson would give Can$1 million for building in return for providing free supplies, in contravention of World Health Assembly Resolutions (Palmer, 1993). The hospital administration overruled the professionals' ethical stance. With this combination of harmful practices and commercial pressures, it is not surprising that throughout the world, where women have received care in the formal health sector, they are least likely to practise optimal breastfeeding patterns (WHO, 1993). Health care systems have damaged breastfeeding.

Throughout the years of breastfeeding decline many women escaped the 'advice' and suckled their babies, as humans had done for thousands of years. The woman who "didn't have no bottle" (Chamberlain, 1983), lived and gave birth in a remote rural area far from hospitals and health visitors. She later (she was interviewed in the 1970s) came to see herself as ignorant and the bottle as progress, but her children survived poverty. She carried the unconscious knowledge of breastfeeding skills from her family culture. She and her friends breastfed on demand because no one had suggested any other way. Their mothers, sisters, and menfolk took it for granted that a baby had to be suckled when it cried. Work and breastfeeding patterns were integrated, just as they are today in the few remaining societies where Western influences have not penetrated too deeply. This assumption of the everydayness of breastfeeding was, and is, the greatest means of 'support, protection, and promotion'. This does not mean that there were no individual problems. A baby may have had an undiagnosed illness and could not suckle effectively. Unwanted infants may have been neglected. What is clear is that the great majority of women breastfed without the self-consciousness and anxiety that is ubiquitous today.

What does all this history-telling have to do with the role of the midwife in breastfeeding promotion? Simply, to understand the source of a problem is the first step to reach its solution. Awareness of how the harmful practices became established helps stimulate the creativity needed for change. There have been many benefits from modern health knowledge, but the development of artificial infant feeding has destroyed a key part of women's power. To reclaim this power we need awareness and clarity about its loss ... and survival.

WHAT IS NECESSARY FOR BREASTFEEDING PROMOTION?

The dictionary definition of 'promote' is to "help forward, encourage, support actively (a cause, process, desired result); to publicize and sell (a product)" (Oxford English Dictionary). For many the promotion of breastfeeding is understood to be achieved through posters and media exhortations about the benefits, and repeated urging of women to breastfeed. However, this appears to be naive and over optimistic. It is useful to analyse the activities of the baby food and feeding utensil companies, who take promotion very seriously indeed. They pay large sums of money to professional experts and advertising and public relations firms to research and implement carefully planned strategies. Yet a small group of health workers and members of mother-support groups are sometimes expected to undertake a breastfeeding promotion campaign with scant resources and no professional consultant to advise them.

There have been successes in breastfeeding promotion through multi-faceted communication campaigns, but they have been co-ordinated, government-led strategies using national and international agency resources and utilizing the skills of promotion professionals. Brazil and Guatemala are examples where, after years of pressure and education by dedicated health professionals and campaigners, the politicians saw the expediency of a co-ordinated breastfeeding campaign. After all, breastfeeding is one of the most cost-effective health interventions and no politician would look bad for promoting it. It is finding the money that tests their commitment. The problem is that no powerful interest group makes an immediate profit from breastfeeding. Governments and health systems will not match the resources of the companies, who invest so much in promotion. For example, in 1990 a British company, Farleys (owned by Boots until 1993, when it was bought by Heinz) spent £3 million (US$4.5 million) promoting one product, Ostermilk (*Chemist and Druggist,* 1991).

Company promotion also works because behind the more overt publicity there is an efficient distribution and public relations' machine that makes those involved feel valued and important. Everyone, from storekeeper to hospital manager, receives something from the system; it may be money, equipment, career advancement, or simply personal attention. Undervalued, overworked health professionals may be taken more seriously by a company representative, may be given some information, a favour, or a gift that makes them feel linked to that person. On a grander scale, there are gifts of equipment, sponsorship for conferences and research grants, endowments, and the underwriting of entire organizations. The established links are so entrenched, so bound up with career progress, so much part of our lives, that whenever implementation of the WHO/UNICEF *International Code of Marketing of Breast-milk Substitutes* [*The Code* (WHO/UNICEF, 1981)] is discussed, there is resistance because of the alleged 'usefulness' of the companies.

What are the rewards for breastfeeding? The obvious answer is a healthy human being, but who acknowledges that? It depends on the society, but certainly gifts and career advancement do not figure, either for the mother or the health professional. For most women, breastfeeding is something they must fit in alongside many obligations to work and family. In many societies women suffer active discrimination for breastfeeding; they are not provided with facilities and are forbidden to bring their babies to work. Is any mother paid to breastfeed? There is no familiar international imagery glamorizing breastfeeding in everyday media. Women in television advertisements promoting other products are never seen breastfeeding. There is no cap and gown or framed diploma.

So, too, for the health professionals; those who dedicate their careers to breastfeeding know that they will not gain the prestige that their colleagues in virology or genetics may gain. If a researcher develops a vaccine, a manufacturer is going to produce it and make money, so there is an immediate motive for financial support. Breast milk and breastfeeding is as powerful and effective as a vaccine and far cheaper, but it is there already and no company or individual is going to become rich from its promotion.

Despite this situation, many dedicated people devote their working lives to the promotion, protection, and support of breastfeeding, because they appreciate the wide-ranging health and social benefits. Many midwives have chosen their career because the personal fulfilment of helping another woman is more important than public glory. However, it is vital to be assertive about the value of breastfeeding and the midwife's work. Those in power who disregard breastfeeding, its value, and the midwife's in supporting it, will not be enlightened unless they are educated. This was the first step in the Brazilian campaign, to raise the awareness of the influential, long before they targeted mothers (WHO/UNICEF, 1981). Midwives, because of their unique closeness to women, can speak with more authority than can other professionals. The midwife's role as a protector of mothers and babies does not end at the bedside. Indeed if she and her representatives neglect the issues of protection in society at large, her more intimate role will be undermined.

It is unfair to urge women to breastfeed while at the same time permitting the pressures to bottle feed. The experience from Brazil has shown that breastfeeding campaigns can only work while *The Code* is being implemented (Ferreira Rea, 1990). Unless all aspects – unethical marketing, workplace facilities, and systems of social support – are tackled, midwives' work will always be undermined. If *The Code* is implemented and commercial promotion is successfully stopped, sales of breast-milk substitutes fall and incidence and duration of breastfeeding increase. This happened in Brazil, Kenya, and Scandinavia during the 1980s. Midwives cannot challenge these wider issues alone, but through joining forces with others.

AWARENESS OF THE PSYCHOLOGY OF 'SELLING'

We must observe how skilled the companies have been and admit that our breastfeeding encouragement may have lacked the psychological manipulativeness of commercial-product promotion. Some women complain of being pressured to breastfeed and certainly an evangelical or even slightly punitive approach has been taken by some midwives anxious to encourage breastfeeding. Company salespeople would never tell you off, be impolite, or say, "I'm too busy to stop and explain things, you'll just have to get on with it," when asked for some extra information or time. Most health professionals have experienced the blandishments of the baby food or drug companies. Do we make mothers feel that special?

Artificial feeding has been promoted as easy, convenient, the answer to a mother's problems, safe, and scientific. The company conveys an image of caring about the individual mother, or health professional, and her problems. Breastfeeding has been presented as likely to go wrong, unpredictable, and needing will-power and perseverance. Much breastfeeding information refers to sore nipples, insufficient milk, engorgement, and tiredness, as though these are inevitable. The most insidious information is distributed by the baby food companies, but it can also come from well-intentioned sources.

The companies downgrade their rival product, breast milk, while appearing to praise it, appropriating the 'gold standard' of breast milk to sell their products, "The next best thing to mother's milk." At the same time, they subtly depict the method of delivering breast milk (breastfeeding) as an ordeal, by emphasizing the apparent ease of bottle-feeding. An extreme example comes from a United States Mead Johnson discharge pack labelled 'BREAST FEEDING ADMISSION KIT', given to breastfeeding mothers in hospital. It is a pretty and useful bag containing a booklet called *Nursing: The First Two Months*. The 'Survival Guide For The First Week' includes the topics of sore nipples, breast pain, fatigue, and depression; 'The Learning Period: The First Two Months' again includes sore nipples and breast pain, as well as breast infection, breast lumps, overabundant milk, lopsided breasts, and, once more, depression. It does not say that most of these problems are iatrogenic, caused by mismanagement around the birth. Then follows 'Spitting up and Vomiting', 'Refusal to Nurse, Fussiness and Colic', and 'Underfeeding' (Mead Johnson, 1991). After such a list, how many baffled first-time mothers would not turn gratefully to the cute little tin of artificial milk, Enfamil, which has been placed thoughtfully in the pretty bag? The logo shows a contented Mother Rabbit feeding baby Peter Rabbit (*The Code* forbids idealization of bottle feeding – actually, baby rabbits would be most unlikely to survive cows' milk feeds).

The most regrettable aspect of this story is that the booklet was derived from a book cited as *first choice in breastfeeding guides* by the International Lactation Consultant Association (ILCA). ILCA is 'a global association for health professionals who specialize in breastfeeding'. ILCA has tried to raise the profile of breastfeeding by adopting the culture of medicine and by professionalizing support of the mother. The very existence of a 'professional' supporter motivates the expectation from clients for the mystique of complex information. Most North Americans already believe that a doctor is needed to assist every birth; it will be sad if every woman comes to believe she needs professional help in order to breastfeed.

Many midwives are also vulnerable to such notions because in their health institutions they may have seen more problematic cases than easy breastfeeding. Even respected and 'radical' midwifery writers may seem to promote bottle feeding and compromise their health messages, perhaps for fear of alienating the reader who has bottle-fed. One such author states, "It is important for all women to know how to sterilise bottles and mix formula milk" (Flint, 1986, p. 176), but she does not say why. In the special cases when artificial feeding is necessary, the support needed means that a health professional must be at hand to assist with the preparation of a substitute feed at the time that it is needed. To educate all women routinely to sterilize bottles is to endorse the assumption that they may eventually abandon breastfeeding. If a woman is artificially feeding from the start, she will need support and education about preparation after the birth when she is actually feeding the baby. If a breastfeeding mother needs to use a substitute feed, it may be safer, whether she uses her own expressed breast milk or an artificial substitute, to use a cup.

The way we treat women who do not breastfeed is important for breastfeeding promotion. Those who do not breastfeed include:

- Women who cannot for medical reasons, e.g., those with a diagnosis of AIDS (i.e., ill with AIDS, not those known to be HIV positive and well; see Appendix III) or breast cancer.
- Women who have so little confidence that, despite wishing to breastfeed, they cannot survive any difficulty and abandon breastfeeding early.
- Those who are resolved not to breastfeed because of a personal or socially induced resistance.

Most of the last two categories come from industrialized societies and, with the right support, can restart breastfeeding if they change their minds. Emotional support for these women does not mean glossing over the risks of bottle feeding which, whatever the setting, is a censorship of information and therefore unethical.

Another commercial adage to learn from is that good promotion comes from a satisfied customer. Breastfeeding, despite the onslaught it has suffered during the twentieth century, has survived because of its own satisfied customers. First, the babies, who benefit from breastfeeding in so many ways. Second, the mothers – during the 1950s and 1960s, when breastfeeding was declining rapidly throughout the world, the movement 'back' towards breastfeeding was initiated by women. The mother support groups were formed in the face of medical indifference or obstruction to breastfeeding. Women wanted to breastfeed; even before research had proven the benefits, many women sensed it was best and they yearned to be close to their babies.

Women from breastfeeding societies are often astonished to discover how hostile some women from industrialized societies feel towards the very idea of breastfeeding. This hostility arises from a collective misery, derived from ignorance and anger. Women who endured sore nipples and other problems that they were told were inevitable, whose babies screamed with hunger as they were taken off the breast, who never understood what damage had been done to them, naturally told their daughters not to suffer. Midwives then have the obligation to 'sell' breastfeeding through making it a pleasure, not a duty. How can this be done? We suggest that there are three areas where midwives can and should be effective. Through the mothers they support, through caring for themselves and their colleagues, and through society at large.

COUNSELLING SKILLS: THE PERSON IS NOT THE PROBLEM

The dictionary defines a counsellor as an adviser, a person trained to give guidance. During the last decade the skills of 'counselling' have developed and evolved beyond these simple definitions. Counselling is not 'giving a bit of advice', though some advice might be part of the process. The WHO *Breastfeeding Counselling Training Course* describes counselling skills thus (WHO, 1994):

> When a health worker counsels a mother, he or she helps her to overcome
> difficulties in a way that leaves her in charge of her own situation.

The reason for including counselling skills in a discussion of breastfeeding promotion is because counselling is one way *to facilitate women's reclaiming of breastfeeding*. Through medicalization, the process has become the property of medical decision. The very term 'lactation management' implies a disease or a procedure which must be controlled by an expert health professional. This medical approach has harmed breastfeeding, which is not a disease but a human relationship that belongs to a mother and her baby. A health worker has no right to 'manage' this relationship, but she can give support and she can protect that relationship from harm. Thoughtful midwives understand this dynamic between restrained and active assistance of a mother through their experience with the birth process. With breastfeeding there is even less need for active help, but the same need for emotional support, especially at the start. Standing back is just as important as providing appropriate information and practical help.

Since few of us are blessed with the talent to make every contact with another person go smoothly, counselling skills can help us all. According to the WHO (1994) *Breastfeeding Counselling Training Course*, the basic principles are:

- Using helpful non-verbal communication.
- Asking open questions.
- Using responses and gestures that show interest.
- Reflecting back what the mother says.
- Empathizing – showing that they understand how a mother feels.
- Avoiding words which sound judgmental.

A particular culture will influence how these skills are implemented; for example, in the case of non-verbal communication, holding a woman's hand or looking her directly in the eyes is an appropriate non-verbal communication in some societies, but not in others. Gentleness and warmth are always appropriate. What is important is that the first contact should make the woman feel good. The midwife's approach to a mother at their first meeting (ideally when she is pregnant) may make all the difference between turning her on or off breastfeeding. The first step in breastfeeding promotion is to help each woman feel surer of her body and herself; counselling skills can help midwives do this.

Counselling skills can also affect relations with colleagues and, most importantly, help them to think about their own feelings. To be effective, care givers must first care about themselves. This is hard for many health professionals to practise. Many have entered the profession with a sense of wanting to give to others and believe that this means personal sacrifice. The profession of midwifery has been forced to take on the culture of nursing and of hospitals. Most midwives have to cope with unsociable schedules, a lack of support systems for child care, and no workplace facilities for breastfeeding. Many health care systems disregard the personal, emotional, and even physical needs of the health worker. Long hours, snatched meals, and being on constant call contribute to the tradition of heroism which makes it hard for one individual to go home on time, to work at a reasonable pace, or to make rational demands. Midwifery is particularly difficult because babies arrive in their own time and at their own pace. Attempts to influence the timing or pace of birth through unnecessary and often risky interventions have been rightly condemned (WHO, 1985), but the necessity of putting others before oneself can become habitual, even when it is not necessary: midwives can forget to attend to their own needs.

When any health professional colleague, whether peer or senior, reacts with indifference or hostility to the change for better breastfeeding practices, it may be because they are suffering a sense of threat. Counselling skills cannot take away that pain immediately, but they will prevent a 'stand off' situation and help ease the team through change. Setting up a support group with colleagues, perhaps one that mixes the disciplines, can help ease misunderstandings. Some midwives may already have supportive colleagues, family, friendships, or religion to nurture themselves and each other. The point is that every midwife must take steps to care for herself. To paraphrase Caroline Flint, in order to cherish and support women through their experience of childbirth *and breastfeeding*, we need to feel loved and cherished ourselves. We can start the cherishing process by cherishing ourselves (Flint, 1986, op. cit. Chapter 1, Introduction, p. 7).

This cherishing includes the struggle for midwives' rights as mothers. This is important, not only for themselves, but also because, whether they wish it or not, they are models in any community. The most sensitive area of a midwife's feelings about the women in her care is that of her own experiences. Some midwives may have chosen not to have children, but others may have wanted to but could not, and have had to come to terms with this. If the midwife does have children, her own birth and breastfeeding experiences will influence her attitudes. It is not easy for a midwife to help a mother if she herself is suffering from being separated from her own baby because there are no facilities in the workplace or she lives too far away to return home to breastfeed. Many midwives make painful compromises and do not breastfeed their own babies as exclusively or for as long as they wish because their rights have been neglected.

Because of the errors in training, many midwives have 'done all the right things', i.e., followed the textbooks, ended up with the misery of any ensuing problems, and so given up breastfeeding. Their pain may be worse than that for other women. Not only have they endured a sense of letting down their own baby, they have been confronted with the fact that they have been 'doing all the wrong things' and letting down their clients. This is sometimes too hard to bear alone and a natural survival process of the human psyche may come into play – denial. Some health professionals can be hostile, dismissive, or trivializing about the value of breastfeeding; usually such an individual has had an unsatisfactory breastfeeding experience themselves. It is vital to the success of breastfeeding promotion that midwives learn to cope with this delicate situation.

Much can be learned from the lay support groups, such as La Leche League, BUNSO in the Philippines, the Nursing Mothers of Australia, Amningshjelpen, the UK's National Childbirth Trust's Breastfeeding Promotion Group (NCT/BPG), and many others, some linked to International Baby Food Action Network (IBFAN). Some groups began to evolve in the 1950s, 1960s, and 1970s in reaction to the lack of support for breastfeeding within the health system. They not only sought out knowledge and supportive health professionals, but quickly realized that emotional support was a key factor. One of the important principles of several of the lay support groups is that of 'debriefing'. For example, the NCT/BPG makes a more rigorous scrutiny of its trainee voluntary breastfeeding counsellors than most midwifery schools do of their students. An applicant, who must have the experience of breastfeeding her child or children, is asked to review her own feelings and motives for wanting to do this work. With guidance she learns to work through and then put aside her own experiences and not let them influence her support of other mothers. This is difficult, but essential to be an effective counsellor. Her training, which includes reading, seminars, and working alongside qualified counsellors, takes about 2 years. Many organizations provide a system of emotional back-up for the counsellors themselves, so that they obtain the support they need for their work.

STARTING RIGHT

Much damage is done through misguided practices early after birth. This is why the midwife has such a crucial role in breastfeeding promotion, because what happens at birth has a profound effect on breastfeeding. When women receive emotional support during labour, they perceive less pain, need less analgesia, and have a shorter labour. Moreover, the more support in labour, the more significantly successful is the breastfeeding outcome in terms of exclusivity, absence of problems, and relationship with the baby (Kroeger, 1993).

Even with optimal emotional support not all births proceed ideally. It is important to be aware of which interventions are most disruptive to breastfeeding. Lynda Rajan (1994) reviewed the impact on breastfeeding of interventions and provides essential information for all midwives. Caution must be exercised in the decision to use some analgesics, such as pethidine, which have a detrimental effect on breastfeeding. Midwives who meet resistance from colleagues need to seek out the relevant articles and share them. "Midwives develop and share midwifery knowledge through a variety of processes," is part of the *International Code of Ethics for Midwives* (International Confederation of Midwives, 1993).

The Ten Steps (WHO/UNICEF, 1989; see Appendix II, page 19) were developed to make breastfeeding establishment easier. In Oman, where commitment to the BFHI has been strong, health workers have reported how the initiative has eased their workload (UNICEF and Ministry of Health, 1994). There is a heartening account from the experience of a group of BFHI assessors visiting a British hospital. In the UK, bottle-feeding is viewed as a 'cultural practice' and many health workers do not believe this can be changed. Women are offered 'a choice' and about 35% 'plan' to bottle-feed. During this BFHI assessment, a Swedish midwife assessor arrived just as a mother had given birth. She had bottle-fed her other child and planned to bottle-feed this one, but the midwife persuaded her to hold her baby skin to skin and to put the baby to the breast right after the birth. Five months later that mother, labelled the 'bottle-feeding type' and from a 'bottle-feeding culture', was exclusively breastfeeding and loving it (Woolridge, 1994). Biology can override culture. Medical folklore has worked hard to interrupt the spontaneous responses between a mother and her child. Commercial interests have worked hard to maintain the effects, but it is possible to interrupt this trail of damage simply by changing practices at birth.

WHERE DO WE GO FROM HERE?

It has been shown that the establishment and duration of breastfeeding is strongly influenced by practices at and after the birth (RCM, 1991). Midwives, therefore, are the natural guardians of breastfeeding. Many have been betrayed by their training, which came from this Western distortion of a natural process. In all sincerity, teachers have imparted these damaging edicts. There are textbooks for sale all over the world which contain misinformation. It can be frightening to face up to a situation where we must confront mistakes, whether our own or others.

An increase in breastfeeding training is starting to redress this sad situation, but the lack of willingness of governments to commit resources for this investment holds back progress. Thousands of health professionals are still denied access to sound information. How can midwives gain knowledge and skills about breastfeeding? There is still much to discover in our understanding of breastfeeding. Simple texts based on current research-based knowledge are the most useful. We would recommend *Helping Mothers to Breastfeed* by Felicity Savage King (1992), published by AMREF (African Medical and Research Association, Wilson Airport, PO Box 30125, Nairobi, Kenya) and available from the publishers and also from TALC (Teaching Aids at Low Cost, PO Box 49, St Albans AL1 4AX, UK). This book is small, inexpensive, and, although written for Africa, is useful for all countries. Our second suggestion is *Successful Breastfeeding* (RCM, 1991) published by Churchill Livingstone and available to order from book shops in many countries. Again, small and relatively low cost, it explains the best way to achieve successful breastfeeding with every reason backed by a scientific citation. It is an excellent text for midwives to show to doctors who are resisting good practice.

It is important to be cautious. Many standard midwifery, paediatric, and nutrition textbooks contain misleading advice if they are pre-1990, and sadly some remain unrevised. *Myles Textbook for Midwives* had erroneous breastfeeding information up until the 11th edition (Bennet and Brown, 1989). Even though a few industry and industry-funded materials appear plausible, they usually have some subtle sabotage built in to the text and, of course, they are only funded through breastfeeding failure.

For the implementation of training programmes, *Breastfeeding Counselling: A Training Course* (WHO, 1994) and *Breastfeeding: The Technical Basis and Recommendations for Action* edited by Randa J. Saadeh (WHO, 1993) are important materials. The WHO/UNICEF (1981) *International Code of Marketing of Breast-milk Substitutes* is essential for monitoring commercial practices. Discovering the sales figures of breast-milk substitutes in local shops is a useful check of community infant-feeding practices, as is assessing breastfeeding rates at immunization clinics. Liaison with the mother-support organizations, regional UNICEF offices, the BFHI Committee, and IBFAN is vital to maintain awareness of both local and distant trends. Events in other regions may have a significant effect. For example, thanks to pressure from Consumer Organizations, the European Community brought in regulations concerning the export of breast-milk substitutes.

The role of the midwife in breastfeeding promotion depends on the individual circumstances of her work. Not to impede is the first rule of professional help to the mother, so the midwife needs to find ways to become highly competent in the knowledge and skills of breastfeeding support. Helping with the establishment of happy breastfeeding for all clients will make a significant step towards promotion. Midwives have the knowledge and experience to be advocates for breastfeeding. Influencing the powerful to make the social changes needed, the workplace facilities, *The Code* implementation, and control of the baby food and bottle companies is possible. No one can work alone, but together, with the armour of knowledge and the authority of experience, midwives can make a difference.

APPENDIX I
The Innocenti Declaration on the protection, promotion, and support of breastfeeding

Recognizing that:
Breastfeeding is a unique process that:
- *provides ideal nutrition for infants and contributes to their healthy growth and development;*
- *reduces incidence and severity of infectious diseases, thereby lowering infant morbidity and mortality;*
- *contributes to women's health by reducing the risk of breast and ovarian cancer, and by increasing the spacing between pregnancies;*
- *provides social and economic benefits to the family and the nation;*
- *provides most women with a sense of satisfaction when successfully carried out; and that:*

Recent research has found that:
- *these benefits increase with increased exclusiveness [no other drink or food is given to the infant; the infant should feed frequently and for unrestricted periods] of breastfeeding during the first 6 months of life, and thereafter with increased duration of breastfeeding with complementary foods, and*
- *programme interventions can result in positive changes in breastfeeding behaviour.*

The Innocenti Declaration was produced and adopted by participants at the WHO/UNICEF policymakers' meeting on 'Breastfeeding in the 1990s: A Global Initiative', co-sponsored by the United States Agency for International Development (USAID) and the Swedish International Development Authority (SIDA), held at the Spedale degli Innocenti, Florence, Italy, 30th July to 1st August 1990. The Declaration reflects the content of the original background document for the meeting and the views expressed in group and plenary sessions. It is available from UNICEF, 3 United Nations Plaza, New York.

WE THEREFORE DECLARE

As a global goal for optimal maternal and child health and nutrition, all women should be enabled to practise exclusive breastfeeding from birth to 4–6 months of age. Thereafter, children should continue to be breastfed, while receiving appropriate and adequate complementary foods, for up to 2 years of age or beyond. This child-feeding ideal is to be achieved by creating an appropriate environment of awareness and support so that women can breastfeed in this manner.

Attainment of the goal requires, in many countries, the reinforcement of a 'breastfeeding culture' and its vigorous defence against incursions of a 'bottle-feeding culture'. This requires commitment and advocacy for social mobilization, utilizing to the full the prestige and authority of acknowledged leaders of society in all walks of life.

Efforts should be made to increase women's confidence in their ability to breastfeed. Such empowerment involves the removal of constraints and influences that manipulate perceptions and behaviour towards breastfeeding, often by subtle and indirect means. This requires sensitivity, continued vigilance, and a responsive and comprehensive communications strategy, involving all media and addressed to all levels of society. Furthermore, obstacles to breastfeeding within the health system, the workplace, and the community must be eliminated.

Measures should be taken to ensure that women are adequately nourished for their optimal health and that of their families. Furthermore, ensuring that all women also have access to family planning information and services allows them to sustain breastfeeding, and avoid shortened birth intervals that may compromise their health and nutritional status, and that of their children.

All governments should develop national breastfeeding policies and set appropriate national targets for the 1990s. They should establish a national system for monitoring the attainment of their targets, and they should develop indicators such as the prevalence of exclusively breastfed infants at 4 months of age.

National authorities are further urged to integrate their breastfeeding policies into their overall health and development policies. In so doing they should reinforce all actions that protect, promote, and support breastfeeding within complementary programmes, such as prenatal and perinatal care, nutrition, family planning services, and prevention and treatment of common maternal and childhood diseases. All health care staff should be trained in the skills necessary to implement these breastfeeding policies.

Operational targets
All governments by the year 1995 should have:

- Appointed a national breastfeeding co-ordinator of appropriate authority, and established a multi-sectoral national breastfeeding committee composed of representatives from relevant government departments, non-governmental organizations, and health professional associations.
- Ensured that every facility providing maternity services fully practices all of the *Ten Steps to Successful Breastfeeding* set out in the WHO/UNICEF (1989) statement *Protecting, Promoting and Supporting Breastfeeding: The Special Role of Maternity Services.*
- Taken action to give effect to the principles and aim of all articles of the *International Code of Marketing of Breast-milk Substitutes* and subsequent relevant World Health Assembly resolutions in their entirety.
- Enacted imaginative legislation protecting the breastfeeding rights of working women and established means for its enforcement.

We also call upon international organizations to:

- Draw up action strategies for protecting, promoting, and supporting breastfeeding, including global monitoring and evaluation of their strategies.
- Support national situation analyses and surveys and the development of national goals and targets for action.
- Encourage and support national authorities in planning, implementation, monitoring, and evaluating their breastfeeding policies.

APPENDIX II
UNICEF and WHO Ten Steps to Successful Breastfeeding
Every facility providing maternity services and care for new-born infants should :

1. Have a written breastfeeding policy that is routinely communicated to all health care staff.
2. Train all health care staff in skills necessary to implement this policy.
3. Inform all pregnant women about the benefits and management of breastfeeding.
4. Help mothers to breastfeed within half-an-hour of birth.
5. Show mothers how to breastfeed and how to maintain lactation even if they should be separated from their infants.
6. Give new-born infants no food or drink other than breastmilk, unless *medically* indicated.
7. Practise rooming-in – allow mothers and infants to remain together 24 h a day.
8. Encourage breastfeeding on demand.
9. Give no artificial teats or pacifiers (also called dummies or soothers) to breastfeeding infants.
10. Foster the establishments of breastfeeding support groups and refer mothers to them on discharge from the hospital or clinic.

From *Protecting, Promoting and Supporting Breastfeeding: The Special Role of Maternity Services.* A joint WHO/UNICEF statement (WHO/UNICEF, 1989).

APPENDIX III
Consensus Statement From The WHO/UNICEF Consultation On HIV Transmission and Breastfeeding, Geneva, 30th April, 1992

RECOMMENDATIONS

1. In all populations, irrespective of HIV infection rates, breastfeeding should continue to be protected, promoted, and supported.
2. Where the primary causes of infant deaths are infectious diseases and malnutrition, infants who are not breastfed run a particularly high risk of dying from these conditions. In these settings, breastfeeding should remain the standard advice to pregnant women, including those who are known to be HIV-infected, because their baby's risk of becoming infected through breast milk is likely to be lower than its risk of dying of other causes if deprived of breastfeeding. The higher a baby's risk of dying during infancy, the more protective breastfeeding is, and the more important it is that the mother be advised to breastfeed. Women living in these settings whose particular circumstances would make alternative feeding an appropriate option might wish to know their HIV status to help guide their decision about breastfeeding. In such cases, voluntary and confidential HIV testing, accompanied in all cases by pre- and post-test counselling, could be made available where feasible and affordable.
3. In settings where infectious diseases are not the primary causes of death during infancy, pregnant women known to be infected with HIV should be advised not to breastfeed, but to use a safe feeding alternative for their babies. Women whose infection status is unknown should be advised to breastfeed. In these settings, where feasible and affordable, voluntary and confidential HIV testing should be made available to women, along with pre- and post-test counselling, and they should be advised to seek such testing before delivery.
4. When a baby is to be artificially fed, the choice of substitute feeding method and product should not be influenced by commercial pressures. Companies are called upon to respect this principle in keeping with the *International Code of Marketing of Breast-milk Substitutes* and all relevant World Health Assembly resolutions. It is essential that all countries give effect to the principles and aim of the *International Code*. If donor milk is to be used, it must first be pasteurized and, where possible, donors should be tested for HIV. When wet-nursing is the chosen alternative, care should be taken to select a wet-nurse who is at low risk of HIV infection and, where possible, known to be HIV-negative.
5. HIV-infected women and men have broad concerns, including maintaining their own health and well-being, managing their economic affairs, and making future provision for their children, and therefore require counselling that includes infant feeding practices, the risk of HIV transmission to the offspring if the woman becomes pregnant, and the transmission risk from or to others through sexual intercourse or blood. All HIV-infected adults who wish to avoid child-bearing should have ready access to family planning and information services.
6. In all countries, the first and overriding priority in preventing HIV transmission from mother to infant is to prevent women of child-bearing age from becoming infected with HIV in the first place. Priority activities are (a) educating both women and men about how to avoid HIV infection for their own sake and that of their

future children; (b) ensuring their ready access to condoms; (c) providing prevention and appropriate care for sexually transmitted diseases, which increase the risk of HIV transmission; and (d) otherwise supporting women in their efforts to remain uninfected.

REFERENCES

Barker, D.J.P. and Osmond, C. (1986) Infant mortality, childhood nutrition and ischemic heart disease in England and Wales. *Lancet*, **i**: 1077–1081.

Barnett, S.A. (1986) Stepney Visitors' Association Report, Oct. 1906–Oct. 1907. Reproduced in *Health Visitor Journal*, Anniversary supplement, September 1986, **59** (9).

Bennet, V.R. and Brown, L.K. (eds) (1989) *Myles Textbook for Midwives*, 11th edn. Churchill Livingstone, London.

Bitoun, P. (1994) Valeur economique de l'allaitement maternel. *Les Dossiers l'Obstetrique*, **216**: 10–13.

Briend, A., Wojtyniak, B., and Rowland, M.G.M. (1988) Breastfeeding, nutritional state and child survival in rural Bangladesh. *British Medical Journal*, **296**: 879–882.

Brock, K.E., Berry, G., *et al.* (1989) Sexual, reproductive and contraceptive risk factors for carcinoma-in-situ for the uterine cervix in Sydney. *Medical Journal of Australia*, **150**: 125–130.

Cadogan, W. (1748) *An Essay upon Nursing and the Management of Children, from their Birth to Three Years of Age*. John Knapton, London.

Carson, C. (1992) Personal communication: Ms Carson (Infant Feeding Supervisor, Birmingham Maternity Hospital, UK) personally supervised the support of the mothers of two sets of breastfed quadruplets – the duration of breastfeeding was 8 months.

Chamberlain, M. (1983) *Fenwoman: A Portrait of Women in an English Village*. Routledge and Kegan Paul, London (first published Virago in 1975).

Chemist and Druggist (1991) Community Pharmacy Supplement, 19 October.

Davies, H.A., Clark, J.D.A., *et al.* (1989) Insulin requirements of diabetic women who breastfed. *British Medical Journal*, **298**(24): 1357–1358.

Davis, M.K., Savitz, D.A., and Graubard, B.I. (1988) Infant feeding and childhood cancer. *Lancet*, **ii**(8607): 365–368.

Elia, I. (1985) *The Female Animal*. Oxford University Press, Oxford.

Facione, N. (1990) Otitis media: an overview of acute and chronic disease. *Nurse Practitioner*, **15**: 11–22.

Fallot, M.E., Boyd, J.L., and Oski, F.A. (1980) Breastfeeding reduces incidence of hospital admissions for infections in infants. *Pediatrics*, **65**: 1034–1036.

Ferreira Rea, M. (1990) The Brazilian National Breastfeeding Programme: a success story. Proceedings from the Interagency Workshop on Health Care Practices Related to Breastfeeding, 1988. *International Journal of Gynaecology and Obstetrics*, **31** (Suppl. 1).

Fildes, V. (1986) *Breasts, Bottles and Babies*. Edinburgh University Press, Edinburgh.

Flint, C (1986) Breastfeeding. In *Sensitive Midwifery*. Butterworth-Heinemann.

Hahn-Zoric, M., Fulconis, F., *et al.* (1990) Antibody responses to parenteral and oral vaccines are impaired by conventional and low protein formulas as compared to breastfeeding. *Acta Paediatrica Scandinavia*, **79**: 1137–1142.

Howie, P.W., Forsyth, J.S., *et al.* (1990) Protective effect of breastfeeding against infection. *British Medical Journal*, **300**(6716): 11–16.

Huggins, K. (1991) *The Nursing Mother's Companion*. Harvard Common Press, Boston.

International Confederation of Midwives (1993) *Code of Ethics for Midwives*. ICM, London.

Jelliffe, Derrick, B. and Jelliffe, E.F. Patrice (1978) *Human Milk in the Modern World.* Oxford University Press, Oxford, p. 237.

Karolinska Institute (1991) *Breastfeeding: The Baby's Choice.* Film. The Karolinska Institute, Stockholm.

Kelly, M. (1993) Infant feeding in emergencies. *Disasters,* **17**(2): 110–121.

King, Sir Frederick Truby (1913) *The Feeding and Care of Baby,* Royal New Zealand Society for the Health of Women and Children. Later edn, 1940, Whitcombe and Tombs, Christchurch, New Zealand.

King, J. and Ashworth, A. (1987a) *Changes in Infant Feeding Practices in Malaysia.* Occasional Paper No 7, Department of Human Nutrition, London School of Hygiene and Tropical Medicine, London.

King, J. and Ashworth, A. (1987b) *Changes in Infant Feeding in the Caribbean,* Occasional Paper No 8, Department of Human Nutrition, London School of Hygiene and Tropical Medicine, London.

Koletzko, S., Sherman, P., *et al.* (1989) Role of infant feeding practices in development of Crohn's disease in childhood. *British Medical Journal,* **2998**: 1617–1618.

Koplick, H. (1903) *The Diseases of Infancy and Childhood.* Henry Kimpton, London, pp 52–53.

Kroeger, M. (1993) Labor and delivery practices: the eleventh step to successful breastfeeding? International Confederation of Midwives, *Proc. 23rd Int. Congress: Midwives Hear the Heartbeat of the Future,* **II**: 1023–1037.

Labbock, M.H. and Hendershot, G.E. (1987) Does breastfeeding protect against malocclusion? An analysis of the 1981 Child Health Supplement to the National Health Interview Survey. *American Journal of Preventive Medicine,* **3**: 227–232.

Lawrence, R.A. (1994) *Breastfeeding: A Guide for the Medical Profession,* 4th edn. Mosby, St Louis, Chapters 3 and 4.

Lucas, A. and Cole, T.J. (1990) Breast milk and necrotising enterocolitis. *Lancet,* **336**: 1519–1523.

Lutter, C. (ed.) (1990) *Towards Global Breastfeeding.* Institute for Reproductive Health (Institute Issues Report), Georgetown University, Washington, DC.

Mayer, E.J., Hamman, R.F., *et al.* (1988) Reduced risk of IDDM among breastfed children. *Diabetes,* **37**: 1625–1632.

Mead Johnson (1991) *Nursing: The First Two Months, A Survival Guide.* From Huggins, K., *The Nursing Mother's Companion,* Harvard Common Press, Boston.

Merrett, T.G., Burr, M.L., *et al.* (1988) Infant feeding and allergy: 12 month prospective study of 500 babies born in allergic families. *Annals of Allergy,* **61**: 13–20.

Ministry of Health (1942) *Report of Advisory Committee on Mothers and Young Children on the Breastfeeding of Infants.* Public Health and Medical Subjects, nos. 88–94, Ministry of Health, London.

Mitchell, E.A., Scragg, R., *et al.* (1991) Cot death supplement: results from the first year of the New Zealand cot death study. *New Zealand Medical Journal,* **104**: 71–76.

Morse, J.M., Jehle., and Gamble, D.(1990) Initiating breastfeeding: a world survey of the timing of post-partum breastfeeding. *International Journal of Nursing Studies,* **27**(3): 303–313.

Oakley, A. (1984) *The Captured Womb: A History of the Medical Care of Pregnant Women.* Basil Blackwood, Oxford.

Palmer, G. (1993) *The Politics of Breastfeeding.* Pandora, London.

Piscane, A., Graziano, L., and Zona, G. (1990) breastfeeding and urinary tract infection. *Lancet,* **336**: 50.

Prentice, A.M., Paul, A.A., *et al.* (1986) Cross-cultural differences in lactational performance. In: Hamosh, M. and Goldman, A. (eds), *Human Lactation 2. Maternal and Environmental Factors.* Plenum Press, London.

Public and General Act (1902) The Midwives Act.

Radford, A. (1992) *Breast Milk: A World Resource.* World Alliance for Breastfeeding (WABA), Penang.

Rajan, L. (1994) The impact of obstetric procedures and analgesia/anaesthesia during labour and delivery on breastfeeding. *Midwifery,* **10**: 87-103.

RCM (1991), *Successful Breastfeeding,* Churchill Livingstone, London.

Riordan, J. and Auerbach, G.K. (1993) *Breastfeeding and Human Lactation.* Jones and Bartlett, Boston, pp 19–20.

Rogan, W.J. and Gladen, B.C. (1993) Breastfeeding and cognitive development. *Early Human Development,* **31**: 181–193.

Rohde, J.E. (1982) Mother milk and the Indonesian economy: a major national resource. *Journal of Tropical Paediatrics,* **28**(4): 166–174.

Savage King, F. (1992) *Helping Mothers to Breastfeed,* AMREF, Nairobi, Kenya.

UK National Case-Control Study Group (1993), Breastfeeding and risk of breast cancer in young women. *British Medical Journal,* **307**: 17–20.

UNICEF (1992) *The Fabella Experience.* Film. UNICEF, New York.

UNICEF and Ministry of Health, Sultanate of Oman (1994) *The Baby Friendly Hospital Initiative, Results from Commitment.* UNICEF and Ministry of Health, Sultanate of Oman, Muscat, pp 23–24.

Victora, C.G., Smith, P.G., *et al.* (1989) Infant feeding and deaths due to diarrhea. *American Journal of Epidemiology,* **129**: 1032–1041.

WHO (1985), *Report on Appropriate Technology for Birth.* World Health Organization, Copenhagen.

WHO (1993) *Breastfeeding: The Technical Basis and Recommendations for Action.* WHO Technical Report P50, World Health Organization, Geneva.

WHO (1994) *Breastfeeding Counselling: A Training Course.* Update No. 14, Division of Diarrhoeal and Acute Respiratory Disease Control, World Health Organization, Geneva.

WHO/UNICEF (1981) *International Code of Marketing of Breast-milk Substitutes,* World Health Organization, Geneva.

WHO/UNICEF (1989) *Protecting, Promoting and Supporting Breastfeeding: The Special Role of Maternity Services.* A joint WHO/UNICEF statement. World Health Organization, Geneva.

WHO Working Group on Infant Feeding (1991) *Facts about Infant Feeding: Breastfeeding and the Use of Water and Teas.* Issue No. 9, World Health Organization, Geneva.

WHO Working Group on Infant Feeding (1992a) *Facts about Infant Feeding.* Issue No. 1, CDR Division, World Health Organization, Geneva.

WHO Working Group on Infant Feeding (1992b) Breastfeeding and Child Spacing. In: *Facts about Infant Feeding.* Issue No. 2, World Health Organization, Geneva.

Woolridge, M. (1994) Personal communication.

A Case Study from Botswana: The Princess Marina Government Hospital

Dikoloti Virginia Morewane

THE BABY FRIENDLY HOSPITAL INITIATIVE IN BOTSWANA

The Baby and Mother Friendly Hospital Initiative (BMFHI) was introduced in Botswana in 1992, based on the WHO/UNICEF BFHI which focuses on the implementation of *Ten Steps to Successful Breastfeeding* (WHO/UNICEF, 1989) – see Chapter 1, Appendix II, page 19. The overall goal of BMFHI in Botswana is to improve the quality of life for babies and mothers by reducing their levels of morbidity and mortality through the exclusive breastfeeding of infants from birth to 4–6 months of age, and by then using appropriate weaning foods up to 2 years and beyond. BMFHI has provided an opportunity to strengthen child feeding practices and their integration into other child survival strategies, such as immunization, safe motherhood, and other mother and child health and/or family planning (MCH/FP) programmes. Furthermore, it provides a deliberate effort to improve the health of the mother and to focus on her as a subject and no longer merely an object. This is particularly opportune as Botswana is working aggressively at present to reduce the maternal morbidity and mortality. Training of individuals, making supportive legislation, and empowerment of women to breastfeed are some of the activities being undertaken to implement BMFHI. The curricula of different health care disciplines are being strengthened to include more education on breastfeeding and safer motherhood.

BMFHI began in an environment in which many hospitals were already changing previously unsupportive routines, such as bottle-feeding, scheduled feeds, and separation of baby and mother after delivery, to more supportive ones. This case study is an account from one such hospital, and examines how such a change was precipitated in 1984 and how it was managed.

TRADITIONAL TSWANA CULTURE

Botswana is a land-locked country bordered by Zambia, Zimbabwe, the Republic of South Africa, and Namibia. It covers an area of $582,000$ km^2 and has a population of 1,330,000. Compared to other countries in Africa, Botswana has relatively low morbidity and mortality rates for children and mothers. Most of the population (86%) has access to health services and 65% of children are fully immunized. The under-five malnutrition rate is 15%. The infant mortality rate is $37/1000$ live births, while the under-five mortality rate is $56/1000$ live births. The maternal mortality rate is $200–313/100,000$ live births.

In Botswana, as in many other African countries, breastfeeding is practised widely and well into the second year of life and beyond. In the traditional Tswana family, the birth of a new baby for a couple strengthens the marital bond and acceptability into the new home for the incoming groom. The newly delivered mother is given the necessary emotional, social, and practical support by the family, especially during the lying-in period (*Botsetsi*), which can last for up to 3 months. During this period routine household chores, like the drawing of water, collecting wood, cooking, and care of other siblings, are done by other family members. Normally, an older member of the family (grandmother or aunt) specially takes care of the newly delivered mother. All the new mother is expected to do is to look after herself and the baby and to eat plenty of food so that she can produce enough breast milk. The breasts are not hidden, and she breastfeeds on demand.

After the lying-in period, the mother is still treated in a special way, so that she can maintain her lactation and care for the baby. The baby may be carried on the mother's back, for instance, on the way to the farm, still be breastfed while she attends to other business, and thereafter sleep over the breast for warmth and comfort.

To make sure that this practice is maintained, some cultural taboos are in force to protect the well-being of both the baby and the mother. Food cooked in a special pot for the new mother can never be shared by other family members, not even the husband. Postpartum abstinence is practised traditionally until the child reaches the age of 1–2 years, but some mothers, especially those in the urban areas, now abstain for shorter periods and then use other family planning methods. During pregnancy, the women receive some special care, such as rest, and are expected to eat plenty for the sake of the baby. The government, too, has instituted supportive policies for pregnant and breastfeeding women, such as the 'breastfeeding hour' (official time off granted to the nursing mother to go and breastfeed her baby) for nursing mothers for the first year postpartum, which came into force in 1984, and the 84 days' fully paid maternity leave for civil servants, which began in 1993.

UTILIZATION OF MATERNAL HEALTH AND FAMILY PLANNING SERVICES

According to the Botswana Family Health Survey (BFHS) of 1988 (Lesetedi *et al.*, 1989), 92% of pregnant women attended antenatal care (ANC) at least once. In urban areas, the percentage of women who attended ANC was 97%, and 91% in rural areas. The MCH/FP programme evaluation in 1989 found the overall use of the ANC service to be 93%, and ANC records in health facilities showed the average number of ANC visits to be five. However, the survey also showed that some high-risk factors, such as pre-eclampsia and previous poor fetal outcome, etc., were not being managed adequately.

The BFHS also found that 77.5% of births during the previous 5 years had been attended by either a nurse-midwife or a doctor, 9% by a traditional birth attendant (TBA), 10% by a relative, while 2% delivered alone. In general, then, the coverage of antenatal care and supervised delivery in Botswana is very good. The health care providers have many opportunities to direct the successful outcome of the service they provide, and to give education on breastfeeding and its management.

Available research shows that breastfeeding practice has declined globally, especially since World War II. Technological advances and Western norms have eroded a noble practice, by manufacturing infant formula as a breast-milk substitute for babies of working mothers. Since then, breast-milk substitutes have been used extensively, for different reasons, in both the developed and developing worlds.

Lamentably, in Botswana, too, breastfeeding practice has declined. According to BFHS II (Lesetedi *et al.*, 1989), breastfeeding declined from 98% to 91% between 1984 and 1988. This decline was sharpest in urban areas, where the mean duration of breastfeeding is 15 months compared to 20 months in rural areas. An International Planned Parenthood Report (IPPF, 1990) also showed that by 4 months after the birth, only 37% of mothers in Botswana exclusively breastfed their children. The Expanded Programme of Immunisation (EPI) KAP (knowledge, attitude, and practice) survey of 1990 also showed that 84% of health care providers knew the benefits of breastfeeding, but that they lacked knowledge of physiology and lactation management (Ministry of Health/UNICEF/WHO, 1990). Of the health care providers interviewed, 37% did not know what stimulates milk supply, and only 8% associated breastfeeding with child spacing.

Some of the most common reasons for this decline in breastfeeding practice are:

• Aggressive marketing and the availability of breast-milk substitutes make women doubt the superiority of their own breast milk.
• The rural–urban migration. Many women, especially the young ones, move away from their families and relatives in the rural areas in search for work. This denies them the sociocultural, psychological, economic, and practical family support that is so crucial to the success of breastfeeding.
• Unsupportive health care practices. Negative attitudes and unsupportive routines of heath care providers, such as giving pre-lacteal feeds to new-born babies and separating baby and mother after delivery, undermine the mother's ability to breastfeed successfully by delaying the onset of lactation.

IMPLICATIONS OF THE DECLINE IN BREASTFEEDING

The decline in breastfeeding results in an increase in infant and maternal morbidity and mortality. The United Nations Children's Fund (UNICEF) estimates that every day between 3000 and 4000 infants die from diarrhoea and acute respiratory infections because the ability to breastfeed them adequately has been taken away from their mothers. Thousands more become victims of other illnesses, malnutrition, and impaired growth and development.

To reverse this serious trend, UNICEF and WHO made some resolutions at the World Health Assembly and other UN meetings which have been adopted for implementation by the different respective national governments.

The 1989 WHO/UNICEF joint statement (WHO/UNICEF, 1989) calls for the protection, promotion, and support of breastfeeding by implementing ten steps to successful breastfeeding in all maternity units. *The Innocenti Declaration* (UNICEF, 1990) (see Chapter 1, Appendix I, pages 17–18) requires that all women should be enabled to practise exclusive breastfeeding from birth to 4–6 months of age, and this be complemented with an appropriate weaning diet for 2 years and beyond. The World Summit for Children requires that women should have the necessary information and environment to breastfeed their infants. The Convention on the Rights of Children, also in 1990, states that children must have the right to be breastfed and the mother too has the right to breastfeed the child. Finally, BFHI aims at protecting the lives of millions of infants by making breastfeeding supported all over the world and improving the status of women in society by empowering them with the information and practical skills that would make them self-sufficient in the care, nutrition and development of their children.

THE PRINCESS MARINA HOSPITAL

The Princess Marina Hospital in Gaborone (the capital city) is a national referral hospital and, indeed, until 1983 it was the only one. It serves as a clinical area for the Institute of Health Sciences, which trains midwives and other health disciplines for the country.

The old system

During the antenatal period, different topics that promote the health of the baby and the mother were introduced to women. The topics were many and all competed for priority. They included, for example, nutrition during pregnancy, breastfeeding, signs of pre-eclampsia, and other indicators of risk and complications. This situation, compounded by the health care providers' lack of knowledge of breastfeeding management, may not have adequately prepared the mother to manage breastfeeding problems.

The maternity section in Princess Marina was divided into Admission and Labour, Puerperium, Ante-Natal Ward, Normal Nursery, Premature Nursery, and the Milk Room. It was a very busy unit with a bed capacity of 37 and yearly deliveries of around 3570 babies. Once a woman had been admitted into Admission and Labour, she would be kept there for 1 h after delivery and, after fourth stage, she would be moved to Puerperium. An already parous woman who delivered normally would usually be discharged within 24 h because of the shortage of space.

After a normal delivery at full term, each baby was taken to the normal nursery to rest for 2 h. They would then be given an initial bath and be passed to their mothers for feeding. If the ward was too busy, the initial bath could be delayed. Feeds were scheduled to be 4-hourly. All mothers were issued automatically with bottles of glucose water initially, and then with infant formula to feed their babies, because 'breast milk was not yet established'. All mothers were encouraged to put their baby to the breast before giving any artificial feed, but were not necessarily given practical assistance by nurses. When

27

lactation was well-established, it was expected that the babies would no longer need the formula. Nurses checked to ascertain that mothers had enough breast milk.

Babies in the Premature Nursery were fed on the prescribed schedule using nasogastric tubes, feeding bottle, or breast, depending on their condition and weight. Sick full-term and caesarean section babies were also admitted there and fed on this schedule, as the others.

This was the ward routine under which almost all midwives were trained. The preparation of artificial feed was one of the procedures in which student midwives were examined. Indeed, the author was trained in this way and accepted and practised this routine without any question.

The catalyst

In 1984, I worked in the MCH/FP clinic adjacent to the maternity ward. On one of my regular visits to the maternity ward, I found that there were many babies sick with diarrhoea and oral thrush in the Premature Nursery. The nursery was so full that some of the sick babies were even in the main ward with their mothers. There was also much overcrowding in the Puerperium Ward because mothers were waiting for their sick babies to become well and be discharged. Some of the newly delivered mothers who had been discharged were readmitted because their babies, too, had diarrhoea and oral thrush.

Stool analysis could not be performed for all the sick babies with diarrhoea. There was a great pressure of work on the laboratory, which served as both a hospital and a national laboratory, plus the severity of illness in some of the babies necessitated immediate therapeutic intervention. Some of the babies were investigated and their stool results taken as representative of all the others. Such an approach can be considered reasonable in view of the likelihood of cross-infection in a facility using open cots with no isolation facilities. There was consistency of the bacterial isolates, which could be divided into three main categories: coliforms, such as E. coli, Salmonella groups, and Klebsiella and the other nosocomial organisms.

The medical and nursing teams worked around the clock to save the lives of the babies. The domiciliary midwife started to carry oral rehydration treatment sachets in her kit to treat other babies in their homes and referred only the very sick ones to the hospital.

It soon became almost impossible to provide enough sterile feeding utensils for each feeding time in the Milk Room. So many of the babies were treated with gentian violet for oral thrush that almost all the teats turned violet as time went on. There was much human suffering all around, and the environment was very depressing.

Interviews with mothers

Interviews with mothers in the maternity ward revealed that they all bottle-fed their babies on the glucose water and/or formula supplied in the ward. About a half of the mothers said they gave the breast first for just a few minutes, because the milk had not 'come in', and then the bottle last. One-quarter gave the bottle first for the same reason, then offered the breast. The remaining quarter said they had problems in fixing babies to the breast, so gave the bottle until they could master the skill of fixing the babies properly. Some of those mothers who had been readmitted to the ward reported that they had continued both breast and bottle feeding at home. Almost all the mothers saw nothing wrong in using the bottle as well as breastfeeding, because they were taught this practice by the health care providers. Some felt that the baby had to become used to the bottle so that when they went back to work, or had to be out of the house, the baby could be fed in this way.

The situation analysis

After assessing the situation in the ward, I produced the following analysis, identifying a number of factors that had contributed to the current crisis situation.

ROUTINE SEPARATION

Routine separation of baby from mother caused delay in the initiation of breast feeding. Available research (WHO/UNICEF, 1993) showed that the mother who delays breastfeeding initiation after delivery takes longer to lactate and tends to breastfeed for shorter periods compared to those who initiated earlier.

The maternal 'sensitive period' is said to be at its highest during the first 1–2 h after delivery. The mother is very sensitive and loving to her baby, which enhances bonding, and the baby is alert at this time. Keeping the baby and mother apart at this crucial period interferes with this natural process, and mothers seemed to worry a lot during this period of separation. This was clear from questions repeatedly asked by many mothers: "Nurse, my baby should be hungry by now", or "Nurse, the baby crying in there is probably mine". Such a state of worry or anxiety might easily counteract the release of the milk ejection hormone (oxytocin) as well.

EARLY BOTTLE-FEEDING

Early bottle-feeding not only fills the baby's tummy, but it may also cause nipple confusion. A baby who has been fed with a rubber teat may find it difficult to fix properly on to the human nipple. Lactation is established when the baby fixes well to the nipple and suckles actively. This strong sucking reflex stimulates the secretion of prolactin (the milk secretion hormone), which in turn leads to secretion of oxytocin (the milk ejection hormone). A baby who has either a full tummy or nipple confusion does not stimulate lactation effectively, a situation that may go unnoticed. If this cycle goes on and on, the mother's breasts may engorge, which makes attachment even more difficult. Failure to empty breast milk leads to a reduction in lactation and then to the 'Not enough milk' syndrome. It is very easy and tempting to the mother in this situation to decide to use the bottle, because she 'does not have enough milk'. If infant formula is aggressively marketed and easily available, as is the case in many countries including Botswana, the mother becomes an easy prey.

IMMUNOLOGICAL PROTECTION

Interference with the immunological protection of breast milk occurs with supplementary feeds. At birth the baby's immune system is still immature and so prone to many infections. Colostrum is the baby's first immunization against many of these infections. Both colostrum and breast milk protect the baby against many pathogens, such as polio virus, hepatitis B virus, and *E. coli*, and several staphylococcal and intestinal bacteria which cause severe intestinal, urinary, and other infections. They also quicken the maturation of intestinal lining, thus creating a barrier against invasion by bacteria and allergens. Also of importance is the acid medium of the baby's stomach, which inhibits growth of harmful bacteria. Any feed at this age that is not breast milk, even if given only once, interferes with these natural defence mechanisms.

The stools from the hospital showed that the babies had ingested some harmful bacteria, probably through feeding bottles. It could be that both mothers and health care providers played a role in the transmission of the infection. Furthermore, poorly sterilized feeding utensils and the overcrowding of mothers and babies, which can give an unhygienic environment, may have contributed. The early introduction of artificial feed using the bottle resulted in the early introduction of harmful bacteria that overpowered the babies' immune systems and resulted in episodes of diarrhoea and oral thrush.

MOTHERS' CONFIDENCE

The undermining of mothers' confidence in their ability to produce enough breast milk for their babies was another by-product of the hospital regime. According to the veteran breastfeeding campaigners, the Jelliffes, lactation is a 'confidence trick'. Failure in healthy well-nourished women with normal full-term babies is most frequently due to the anxiety–nursing–failure cycle – based on emotional interference with the let down reflex (Jelliffe and Jelliffe, 1978). Every effort must be made to empower the mother to feel confident about breastfeeding and to assist her to practise it fully. This makes it mandatory for health care providers to practise what they teach, for otherwise they cause confusion and undermine the mother's confidence in them. They must be seen to whole-heartedly believe in the superiority of breast milk.

Since bottle feeding was 'prescribed' indiscriminately to all babies, mothers did seem obliged to do what everybody was doing without question. Because health care providers did not ask questions or actively offer practical assistance to mothers, they could also miss some of the factors that were hindering successful breastfeeding. This was perhaps unsurprising, because the curricula of different health disciplines provided scanty information to equip a practitioner to protect, promote, and support breastfeeding effectively.

Planning change

With this analysis of the prevailing situation, I felt that there were enough hard facts to mandate an urgent change in order to improve the quality of life and alleviate the human suffering of the babies delivered in Princess Marina. This would, in turn, benefit the well-being of the mother, help to minimize the amount of bleeding in the immediate postpartum period, and help to increase birth intervals if exclusive breastfeeding was established. A problem-solving model for change (Brooten et al., 1978) was used.

Meetings were arranged with different people to discuss the problem at hand. First, I met with the senior nursing sister in charge of the ward, who agreed that there was crisis in her ward and that it needed to be resolved urgently. She was willing to listen to any suggestion that could reverse the situation.

I proposed the following:

• That all babies should be given to their mothers straight after birth, and that all mothers should be assisted practically and supported to breastfeed on demand by the nurses allocated to the Normal Nursery, Milk Room, and Puerperium. Each baby should sleep with his/her mother on the same bed, and no longer in the cot hanging at the foot of the mother's bed. This would encourage early lactation, and facilitate demand feeding and bonding. Mothers needing help would be supported and communication between health care providers and mothers would improve. Mothers might start to believe they do have enough milk and that their milk is superior to artificial feed. Babies, too, would not run the risk of nipple confusion.

- That the initial bath for the babies be delayed to even up to the following day. Among other things, this would facilitate the resting together of baby and mother.
- That babies who, for any reason, cannot breastfeed be fed by cup and spoon on breast milk unless medically indicated. This regime was to be used with both new-born babies and those that were in the ward already. This would stop any chance of nipple confusion, and any unnecessary use of infant formula. The availability of sterile feeding utensils would be maximized and the chances of cross-infection minimized.
- That more up-to-date information of the value of breast milk and how breastfeeding can be protected, promoted, and supported should be given to nurses and other health care providers. This would empower health care providers to support and mothers to practise exclusive breastfeeding from birth up to the first 4–6 months of age, and the probability of continuing for up to 2 years of age and beyond would be maximized.
- That nurses should explain the desired outcome thoroughly to the mothers and should give them the necessary practical help. This would give mothers a chance to make an input in the change process and to prepare them psychologically to participate willingly.
- That the domiciliary midwife follow-up and see if mothers continued breastfeeding exclusively after discharge from hospital.

The ward sister agreed with the suggestions, but wanted to employ an effective strategy that had the potential for good results. She agreed to participate in the change process and that I should spearhead it.

After many questions, a large number of nurses were willing to participate in the process provided they were given enough information and that they had the backing of their supervisors and hospital administration if things did not work out as expected. Some nurses were not willing to participate because they insisted that if the babies were not bottle-fed before their mothers milk 'came in' they would starve. They also argued that babies and mothers needed rest after delivery. They furthermore believed that mothers would refuse to accept babies before the initial bath. They felt it would be seen as laziness on the part of the nurse, and would be culturally unacceptable to the mother. Since they were not convinced themselves, there was no way in which this group of nurses could convince mothers. However, importantly, the two groups of nurses were allowed to attend all planning meetings and they were encouraged to voice their fears. These meetings helped to bring out the real and potential problems that might be encountered in the process.

The proposals were received with mixed feelings by the midwifery tutors, because the change would reduce the number of clinical areas for pupil midwives. They pointed out that previously some students had been examined on the making up of artificial feed, such as glucose water or formula, and the changes would deprive them of this. The tutors also argued that further research was required to prove that the babies would not starve when only breastfed. After some discussions, the ward sister ruled that in the interest of the patients the proposed changes should be carried out.

The Paediatrician and Gynaecologist Obstetrician were agreeable to the proposals, but some of the members of their teams were not thoroughly convinced. Some believed that the babies would become hypoglycaemic because of the small amount of colostrum available on the first day. Since they were not usually involved in the actual feeding of babies they were prepared to wait and see, so long as there was vigilance to ensure that the babies' lives were not in any way endangered.

The matter was also broached with the hospital administration, including the matron. After many questions it was agreed that the suggestions should be given a chance to work. The administrators were happy to hear that the desired change would bring down the hospital's expenditure and improve the quality of life for the baby and the mother.

The mothers in the Antenatal Ward, MCH/FP clinic, and Postnatal Ward were all pleased that they would be given their babies soon after birth. A large number were concerned that their babies might be hungry, and that the nurses must be available to offer artificial feed when the babies cry. Almost all of them believed that babies delivered at home hardly ever needed any artificial feeding. They said that women at home are given plentiful liquids, soft porridge, milk, tea, and other traditional lactagogues, and that they are supported to breastfeed. They believed that if care and support at the hospital could be individualized, as it is at home, the plan would work.

Some mothers believed that babies should be bathed after delivery because they are 'dirty', but when asked to choose between the two priorities – an early breastfeed because of the many benefits or an early bath, they chose breastfeeding. Information on the benefits of breastfeeding was shared with many mothers on regular visits to the clinic. Management of breastfeeding difficulties was discussed also.

Planning meetings with nurses continued. More information on the value of breast milk and management of breastfeeding in general was shared with everybody. Communication skills were revisited. Nurses who were ready to participate in the change process were allocated to strategic areas, such as the Premature Nursery, Puerperium, Labour Ward, and Milk Room, on each shift. A co-operative strategy for change was used, allowing members of the group to state freely their concerns, and individual differences were accepted by all.

Nurses who were not ready to participate were encouraged to voice their fears, and nobody was supposed to pin them down for their opinion. Fortunately, the implementation coincided with the period when pupil midwives were 'on block', which reduced the number of people to deal with, made supervision lighter, and increased the chances of success. Although this process to change the routine seemed to have taken a long time to prepare, it was actually implemented within 2 weeks. The treatment of the sick babies was, of course, also actively carried on while the plans for the change in care were being made.

Implementation: a matter of acting

When the roles of the nurses were clearly defined and the mothers had been informed about the change, the plan was implemented. All the babies delivered were dried and given to the mother straight away. Mothers were assisted to fix the babies to breastfeed whenever there was a need. Breastfeeding was done on demand and mothers were allowed to sleep with their babies. The initial bath was delayed for more than 6 h, or even up to the following day.

The babies who were already in the ward were also breastfed only. The sick and pre-term babies who could not breastfeed were fed on expressed breast milk or, if medically indicated, on artificial feed by cup and spoon.

Both the ward sister and myself were there to participate and/or support the staff and the mothers. Regular meetings to measure progress and to detect any obstacles were held. Meetings were open to all nurses and other health care providers.

Evaluation

On evaluation, we found that there was more success than difficulty. Nurses gave mothers the support and practical help and all of them breastfed their babies. Nurses were available to assist the mother when the baby cried, but babies generally cried less because they were fed on demand, not 4-hourly as before, and were also within easy reach of their mothers for comforting.

Initially, some mothers who were doubtful, especially the private patients who had brought their own bottles and found that they did not even use them. Mothers in the Pre-term Nursery felt it was slow to spoon-feed their infants, but they later mastered the art. As time went on they fed their infants on cup only, without a spoon, and did very well. Some of the mothers who had wished to be given their baby already bathed became more consoled to the benefits of early breastfeeding initiation and they accepted the change.

All the other staff members who did not believe the change would work saw the results and slowly they joined in. There were no new outbreaks of diarrhoea and oral thrush. Mothers did not have their breasts infected with fungus. The domiciliary midwife also confirmed that there were no new outbreaks of diarrhoea or thrush in the newly discharged babies.

She did report, however, that some mothers still introduced the bottle to the baby because they would soon be going back to work. They felt that the babies had to become used to the bottle early (e.g., at 1–2 months of age), in case they refused it later on.

Stabilization

Both the health care providers and mothers accepted the change as the new routine that should be practised by everybody in the ward and at home. The ward sister destroyed the used and new bottles and teats in stock because they were no longer needed.

The hospital administrator was no longer required to order bottles and teats and large stocks of formula, which saved a lot of hospital money. When the pupil midwives came for their clinical work, they found that the new routine was working well and they followed it. This new ward routine was written on the notice board and other target places for everybody to see.

Furthermore, when the ward sister was transferred to another hospital in the country, she introduced the same change and succeeded very well. Also, all the midwifery tutors were supportive of the change and taught the new method to all their midwives. The newly qualified midwives also managed to change bottle-feeding to breastfeeding in different hospitals where they were posted after completion of their studies.

IMPLICATIONS OF THE CHANGE

The overall goal of this change was to reduce the morbidity and mortality of babies and mothers through improved quality of breastfeeding. Since the rampant attacks of diarrhoea and oral thrush in infants were eradicated the change achieved some of its aims in this aspect, and it is hoped that in the long run the overall goal will be achieved. The new written routine on infant feeding served as a standard against which the care given could be measured; this is an important issue. Written nursing standards should be known and practised by all. Health care consumers, too, should have access to such standards as they have the right to know and criticise the care they receive. To back this up, the nursing service should mandate that its practitioners are given pre- and in-service education on a regular basis in order to be safe and up-to-date practitioners. Both the nursing service and nurse education bodies should make arrangements to purchase books and other teaching aids, and to receive literature on breastfeeding from international sources.

RESEARCH NEEDS

As in other health care disciplines, nursing needs much more research into its practice. Breastfeeding is one topic that is poorly researched. It is taken for granted as a natural instinct, but there is an urgent need to research breastfeeding in order to provide the basic information on breastfeeding patterns and factors that influence them, and to guide the implementation of BMFHI. A breastfeeding database should be established in order to provide timely information, and results of the research should be disseminated periodically so as to provide current information on breastfeeding and facilitate self and continuing education.

I would like to encourage midwives and other health care providers to initiate change without fear to improve the standards of the care we give, and I sincerely want to thank the Maternity Ward Sister in charge (Mary-Anne Bale), her staff, and everybody who supported this change.

REFERENCES

Brooten, D., Hayman, L., and Naylor, M. (1978) *Leadership for Change: A Guide for the Frustrated Nurse.* J.B. Lippincott Company, New York.

IPPF (1990) *Survey on Child Survival, Botswana.* International Planned Parenthood.

Jelliffe, D. and Jelliffe, P. (1978) *Human Milk in the Modern World.* Oxford University Press, Oxford.

Lesetedi, L.J., Mompati, D.G., Kulumani, P., Lesetedi, G.N., and Rutenberg, N. (1989) *Botswana Family Health Survey II 1988.* Central Statistics Office, Ministry of Finance and Development Planning, Family Health Division, Ministry of Health, and Institute of Resource Development/Macro Systems, Inc. Colombia, Maryland.

Ministry of Health/UNICEF/WHO (1990) *The Botswana EPI Evaluation.* United Nations, Florence, Italy.

UNICEF (1990) *Innocenti Declaration on the Protection, Promotion, and Support of Breastfeeding.*

WHO/UNICEF (1989) *Protecting, Promoting and Supporting Breastfeeding: The Special Role of Maternity Services.* A joint WHO/UNICEF statement.

WHO/UNICEF (1993) *Breast Feeding Management and Promotion in a Baby Friendly Hospital. A Course for Maternity Staff.* World Health Organization, Geneva.

BIBLIOGRAPHY

Anderson, S. and Staugard, F. (1986) *Traditional Midwives (Traditional Medicine in Botswana).* Ipelegeng Publishers, Gaborone.

Chetley, A. (1979) *The Baby Killer Scandal.* War on Want, London.

Government of Botswana and UNICEF (1993) *Situation Analysis of Children and Women in Botswana.*

Helsing, E. and Savage King, F. (1982) *Breast Feeding in Practice.* Oxford University Press, Oxford.

La Leche League International (1987) *The Womanly Art of Breast Feeding.* Franklin Park, Illinois.

Lanwers, J. and Woessherc, C. (1983) *Counselling the Nursing Mother.* Avery Publishing Group Inc., New Jersey.

Lawrence, R. (1985) *Breast Feeding: A Guide for the Medical Profession.* The CV Mosby Company, Toronto.

Morewane, D.V. (1985) *Role of Health Education in Promotion of Breast Feeding.* Paper presented to first International Conference in Health Education, Harrogate. Unpublished.

Ntombela, N., Morewane, D., and Karamagi, C. (1994) *Report on Strengthening BMFHI in Botswana.* UNICEF, Gaborone.

Safe Motherhood Task Force (1992) *Safe Motherhood in Botswana.* Family Health Division, Ministry of Health, Gaborone.

Savage King, F. (1993) *Helping Mothers to Breast Feed.* African Medical Research Foundation, Nairobi.

Steves, W. (1978) *Management and Leadership in Nursing,* McGraw-Hill, New York.

Williams, C. and Jelliffe, D. (1972) *Mother and Child Health (Delivering the Services).* Oxford University Press, Oxford.

CHAPTER 3

A Case Study from Australia: The Northpark Private Hospital

Suzanne Murray

Australia is a very large continent, with a population that is quite small for such a large land mass. Most people live close to cities around the coastline. The climate varies greatly. In the north it is hot and tropical, but in the south it can become quite cold.

The number of Australia's original inhabitants, the indigenous aborigines, in their traditional society is sadly depleted; they are now mainly located in central Australia. Australians of aboriginal background, for the most part, have lost touch with their rich cultural heritage and live in cities, absorbed in the general population. Like the non-aboriginal population, they too are mostly struggling to retrieve lost breastfeeding knowledge and skills.

Non-aboriginal settlement in Australia is relatively recent, a little over 200 years. Early settlers were mainly from the United Kingdom, later from Europe, and more recently from Asia and South America.

MIDWIFERY IN AUSTRALIA

Midwives in Australia undertake their training in general nursing for 3 years before the 1 year postgraduate course in midwifery. Formerly, these courses were hospital based, but have now been transferred to the higher education sector. Some midwives take their education one step further and study for another year to become qualified to advise and support mothers of babies, infants, and children to 5 years of age. In Victoria they are known as Maternal and Child Health nurses and provide a council-run service of both home visits and well-baby clinic appointments. They monitor the growth and development of infants and children, and provide an invaluable support service for new mothers.

Midwives work in many and varied settings: some in the very isolated outback of Australia, but most in the hospitals and community health centres of cities and towns. Because of Australia's rich cultural mix, midwives need to be knowledgeable about, and sensitive to, the beliefs and customs of many ethnic groups when caring for mothers and babies.

A small number of midwives have ventured into private practice and are specially licensed to give total care for women during pregnancy, birth, and the postpartum period. The greater majority of midwives, however, are obliged to work under the direction of doctors. Most women give birth in hospital.

It had been usual for women to stay in hospital after delivery for a week or more, but with increasing financial constraints on hospital budgets, this period is being greatly reduced. Opinion varies greatly as to the direct effect on breastfeeding outcomes of early discharge.

BREASTFEEDING IN AUSTRALIA

Breastfeeding in Australia declined and reached its worst trough in the late 1960s and early 1970s. This was largely due to the rigid hospital practices and routines detrimental to breastfeeding success, such as separation of the mother and baby, scheduled and timed feeds, and routine supplementation with artificial milk formula. Very few women survived this insult to their lactation. Some managed to struggle on for about 6 weeks, a small percentage breastfed for 3 months, and an even tinier percentage breastfed for 6 months. Many women and babies were let down by the system of the day, and were deprived of the many benefits and pleasures of breastfeeding. These women are the grandmothers of the present day. Many look back on their own experience with great sadness and most are very ill-equipped to be of help and support to their daughters presently trying to establish breastfeeding.

As women lost their breastfeeding skills, so did the midwives. Health professionals became very knowledgeable about the newly fashionable modified cow's milk, known as formula. Too late, it was realized how poor and second rate this alternative was, by which time midwives had lost their skills in breastfeeding support to a significant degree. This becomes quite obvious when the textbooks and curricula of the ensuing years are reviewed. There has been very little time given to the science of lactation and the art of breastfeeding, in both midwifery and medical education.

At present the rate of initiation of breastfeeding in Australia is quite high compared to other industrialized nations, but the rate of duration drops dramatically in the subsequent weeks and months. In the second most populous state, Victoria, 75% of new mothers leave hospital breastfeeding exclusively, but by 3 months only 52.7% are still breastfeeding, and by 6 months this number has dropped to 39%.

Babies are a very important and appealing part of any society, and no less so in Australia. Although Australians thankfully do not suffer the same level of devastating morbidity and mortality due to bottle-feeding as seen in the developing world, the importance of breastfeeding to all babies is understood. Many people, including government bodies, do not wish to sit by and see our Australian infants being deprived of the enormous benefits of breastfeeding and being exposed to the dangers of bottle-feeding. Although the effects of bottle-feeding in an advantaged country are less easily recognized, it is still impossible to ignore current scientific information (Walker, 1993). Misinformed community and health professional perceptions that the choice of infant feeding is an either/or situation which implies equivalence is no longer acceptable.

According to Morrow and Barraclough (1993), breastfeeding has gained a place in the public policy agenda in Australia and its superiority is now universally acknowledged. It is included in Australia's target of *Health for All by the Year 2000*, in which the government aims to increase breastfeeding rates at 3 months to 80%.

Under Australia's federal system, health responsibilities are shared by the Commonwealth, States, and Territories, although it is common for the National Government to play a leading role in seeking to develop national policy initiatives. The government's advisory body is the National Health and Medical Research Council (NH&MRC). The Federal Government must, in most cases, rely on the states for health statistics. Only Victoria's Maternal and Child Health Service still annually collects and publishes breastfeeding statistics. Questions that relate to patterns of morbidity in the infant and child populations can only be answered in very general descriptive terms.

Morrow and Barraclough (1993) also have pointed out that, as in most countries, Australia does not have a formal structure for designing and disseminating breast-feeding policy, although the joint WHO/UNICEF *Innocenti Declaration* of 1990 (see Chapter 1, Appendix I, pages 17–18) calls for the establishment of a national breastfeeding co-ordinating body in all countries. Instead, one must look for references to breastfeeding in policy documents emanating from various official sources.

In 1990, a state government *Ministerial Review of Birthing Services in Victoria* was completed (Health Department of Victoria, 1990), with submissions from breast-feeding mothers and many agencies and groups, including midwives, maternal and child health nurses, and members of the Nursing Mothers' Association of Australia. The report noted the absence of a uniform approach to encouraging and promoting breastfeeding in Victorian hospitals and birthing services. It revealed that inconsistent knowledge, practices, and attitudes among health workers posed problems for new mothers trying to establish breastfeeding.

In response to this a working party was formed, including health professionals and representatives of consumer groups, to develop a uniform protocol for Victoria. The document, *Promoting Breastfeeding* (Victorian Breastfeeding Guidelines, 1994), was widely distributed to midwives, doctors, hospitals, and other agencies who have contact with breastfeeding mothers.

Included in this document are the state-wide 'Principles of Breastfeeding', endorsed by the Breastfeeding Protocol Committee of Victoria. The aim of the principles is to provide and ensure an atmosphere in the Victorian community that is conducive to successful lactation and breastfeeding. The document states that women should have:

- Clear and correct information about the benefits of breastfeeding to themselves, their infants, and their families.
- Support of their decision to breastfeed by their families, their communities, their health care workers, their health care institutions, and their government.
- Education and support which increase their skills and confidence, enabling them to sustain their planned breastfeeding experience.
- Knowledge of, and access to, community support groups which are involved both in antenatal and postnatal breastfeeding support, such as the Nursing Mothers' Association of Australia.

Also, infants should have:

- The opportunity to gain the full health, psychological, and developmental benefits of breast-milk feeding, even if they have to be separated from their mothers.

- The opportunity to be breastfed exclusively for at least the first 6 months of their lives and to continue breastfeeding with the addition of appropriate weaning food for 12 months, 2 years, or beyond according to what is mutually agreeable to mother and child.

Further, midwives and other health care workers should have:

- Lactation education which is current, scientific, factual, and practical.
- Orientation and continuing education which gives, and builds on, skills that equip them to be consistent and constructive in their support of breastfeeding mothers and their infants.
- A working atmosphere which acknowledges and affirms the importance of their role in breastfeeding support.

And, finally, health care institutions should have:

- A written breastfeeding policy which is freely available to both staff and parents.
- Written programmes for orientation, an education curriculum, and quality assurance programmes which demonstrate the implementation of the breastfeeding policy.
- An atmosphere which encourages their employees to increase their lactation knowledge and skills so that each demonstrates a commitment to the policy of the institution.
- A demonstrated commitment to, and a clear understanding of, the principles of the *International Code of Marketing of Breast-milk Substitutes* (WHO/UNICEF, 1981) and the joint WHO/UNICEF statement *Protecting, Promoting and Supporting Breastfeeding: The Special Role of Maternity Services* (WHO/UNICEF, 1989).

THE GLOBAL BABY FRIENDLY HOSPITAL INITIATIVE
The intent and concept of the Baby Friendly Hospital Initiative (BFHI) is very important to Australia and to Australians. There is an obvious increased awareness of the importance of breastfeeding in the community, and particularly in the midwifery and medical fields. This is demonstrated by the increasing numbers of qualified Lactation Consultants. At present there are about 1000 people who have passed the International Board Examination, the first of which was held in Australia in 1985 (aproxomately 200 sit the exam each year). The largest group are midwives and maternal and child health or early childhood nurses. An increasing number of medical practitioners, including paediatricians and obstetricians, have also qualified. The rest are mostly paediatric nurses, mother-craft nurses, and lay counsellors.

Fortunately for Australian babies, since 1964 there has been a very strong lay counselling group, founded by a small group of mothers. Mary Paton and five of her friends started to meet to support one another in their efforts to breastfeed their babies at an historically appalling time for breastfeeding practice. Since then, the Nursing Mothers' Association of Australia (NMAA) has grown to its present membership of 14,000 women all around the country. It is estimated that over these past 30 years more than 120,000 women have been members and countless more breastfeeding women have been helped by the Association. NMAA has borne a very large part of the responsibility for breastfeeding support, which perhaps should have always been the responsibility of governments and health professionals.

As illustrated previously, there is now a very strong government commitment to the promotion, support, and protection of breastfeeding in Australia. BFHI provides a way of encouraging health professionals to look at and evaluate their own practice and, indeed, to take responsibility for their actions.

It provides a structure and a system for health care facilities to gain certification of good practice in breastfeeding, just as they do for many other aspects in the work place, such as policy and procedure for medical and surgical care, occupational health and safety, and staff training and education in their particular specialties.

BFHI gives management and staff a very real incentive to look systematically at all aspects of the care of breastfeeding women and babies. They can then make the changes necessary to achieve the standards that are required to apply for assessment. It provides a very real opportunity for those who have already recognized that change is needed to effect this change in a positive and acceptable form.

In Australia, BFHI is being directed by a National BFHI Authority, formerly known as the BFHI Taskforce and later as the BFHI Steering Group, all overseen by UNICEF. Its members have included representatives of all the major groups who would have any interest or influence in the concept. These include the Australian College of Midwives, the Australian College of Paediatricians, the Australian College of Obstetricians and Gynaecologists, the Directors of Nursing Associations, the College of Hospital Administrators, the Nursing Mothers' Association of Australia, Maternal & Child Health Nurse Association, the Australian Lactation Consultants Association, the College of General Practitioners, the Australian Nursing Federation, Community Aid Abroad, Australian Association of Paediatric Teaching Centres, and the Centre for Mothers' and Children's Health. Recently, a National Co-ordinator has been sponsored by UNICEF. It is expected that BFHI will be self-funding. Workshops have been provided to train assessors and a data bank of these trained assessors has been set up. The National Authority provides policy to assist implementation of the initiative.

HOW TO MAKE YOUR MATERNITY HOSPITAL BABY FRIENDLY

It is very important to understood that the BFHI is not meant to place any pressure on mothers. It is not designed to force mothers to breastfeed. It is designed to be protective of those mothers who choose to breastfeed. It is designed to provide a positive breastfeeding atmosphere for women, in which, in a spirit of encouragement, staff evaluate their own work and practice. The staff aim to improve any short-falls and make a very real commitment to positive change that helps mothers towards the early establishment of breastfeeding.

Initially, you need to show the management of your hospital that there are very positive benefits to both the image and the running of the hospital by its becoming part of the initiative. It is essential to have the backing of senior management, who have the power to make things happen. Management must see the BFHI as attractive to them. Perhaps it may be the aspect of the prestige of being the first, the best, the most innovative. Perhaps there may be definite cost benefits that can be displayed to them.

This is what we have done and are doing at my hospital, Northpark, which is in a suburb about 30 minutes from Melbourne, the capital city of Victoria. Northpark is an 80-bed private hospital which provides midwifery, medical surgical, and psychiatric care. We realize that it is not only important to make our 14-bed midwifery unit baby friendly, but to recognize also the importance to the rest of the hospital, which sometimes admits mothers and babies when the mother is ill.

Start out by finding other staff members who are interested in helping mothers to breastfeed. It is important to form a supportive group when one is trying to change the work place and to change attitudes. This core group needs to be very familiar with the WHO/UNICEF *Ten Steps to Successful Breastfeeding* (see Chapter 1, Appendix II, page 19), with each able to explain the background and intention of each of the ten steps. Colleagues may at first be suspicious of the initiative if they do not totally understand its intention. Once the group is formed, make plans to have a Baby Friendly Initiative Information Night. Include in the invitations senior management, midwifery and medical staff, and auxiliary staff. Do not forget that there are many people who come in contact with breastfeeding mothers during their daily work. It is not just the medical or nursing staff who may make comments and influence mothers. Each staff member has the potential to influence various aspects of the endeavours to make a hospital baby friendly. It is very important to have each informed and included right from the very start. Allies can come from the most unexpected quarters.

When planning for your hospital, use the ten steps and work through them from the start. Use of the ten steps as a basis for all planning of care of breastfeeding women and babies, staff education, procedures, protocols, and written information will also prepare the hospital for later accreditation.

Once you have formed a BFHI supporters' group you may decide to formulate your own written breastfeeding policy, which is totally relevant to your own work place (Murray, 1993), or you may decide to adopt an established local, regional, or government policy. As Step One of the BFHI implies, this policy must be accepted by the medical and nursing staff so a consultative process is ideal. Once ratified the policy must be freely available to both mothers and care givers. Perhaps the policy should be in bed-side folders for the mothers, copies displayed prominently in different work areas, and copies available for loan from formal or informal libraries. Each new staff member should be given their own copy of the breastfeeding policy when being orientated to the hospital.

How to involve the doctors is a very real challenge

In Australia, medical education about breastfeeding has not been comprehensive nor well-organized. There has been little incentive for medical students to value breastfeeding as an important health issue, or to gain any real supportive skills. It is only relatively recently that there have been any examination questions on this topic. It may, therefore, be quite threatening for medical practitioners to be confronted with such issues as policy and procedure when they do not really feel comfortable in their own knowledge. It may be that they have to rely heavily on their own personal or family experiences, which may have been much less than ideal.

They need, however, to read and approve the hospital breastfeeding protocol and to be invited to general breastfeeding education programmes. An individual approach and case discussion may prove to be more effective, or another approach may be to provide audio tapes of education sessions, which can be used at a convenient time and avoid time-consuming reading.

Next, for Step Two, a full education programme is needed to equip the staff with the knowledge and the skills they need to operate fully in a 'baby friendly' mode. Of course, if one is baby friendly it naturally follows that one is mother friendly also.

The education programme needs to have a strong clinical component. The theoretical component needs to be backed up by supportive literature and a reading list. The curriculum needs to include:

- The advantages of breastfeeding and the disadvantages of artificial feeding.
- The anatomy of the breast, changes during pregnancy and lactation, physiology of lactation.
- Techniques for breastfeeding – positioning, attachment (latch-on), feed assessment, milk ejection, milk transfer, pattern of infant sucking.
- The importance of the attitude and encouragement of the midwife, the obstetrician, the paediatrician, and the general practitioner.
- The importance of an early, *effective* first breastfeed, and on-going feed assessment, observation, and support of mother and baby, unrestricted breastfeeds in time, frequency, and duration, the expected output of the baby as a sign of well-being.
- Supportive rooming which encourages access of mother and baby – no unnecessary separation.
- Frequent, effective breast 'emptying', either by direct breastfeeding or by breast expression.
- Expression of the breast by hand, or hand and pump, and care of expressed breast milk.
- Management for maintaining lactation when the infant feeds ineffectively or is unable to feed directly from the breast.
- Avoidance of detrimental practices – complementary or supplementary feeds, artificial sucking objects, endorsement or promotion of artificial feeds.
- Responsibilities to the WHO Code (WHO/UNICEF, 1981).
- Common problems of breastfeeding – sore nipples, damaged nipples, inverted nipples, engorgement, mastitis, prior breast surgery, sleepy baby, jaundiced baby, premature baby, baby with a disability.
- Use of nipple shields, breast shells, and supply line.
- Weaning and natural suppression of lactation.

We have found that the clinical component of staff education is best done in small groups at the mother's bedside. Staff need to observe the individuality of mothers and babies and the different styles and positions they adopt when breastfeeding. The staff need to understand the essential, basic principles of positioning and attachment (latch-on) and how to adapt these to suit individual situations. They must always be aware that the mother is the breastfeeder and that the help given needs to be gentle and unobtrusive. Delivery room staff must be particularly aware of the baby's alert time after birth, and should take care to allow the baby to have access to the breast. The baby should not be pushed to the breast, but allowed to follow the course of pre-feeding behaviour, including mouthing, licking, and tongue thrusting. All staff need to be made aware of and able to observe effective, pain free breastfeeding with good milk transfer.

The antenatal midwife educators share the responsibility for Step Three of the BFHI with the mothers' doctors. They use formal classes to teach all pregnant women about the benefits and management of breastfeeding. Prior to this, when booking into the hospital, the couple should have time with a midwife to discuss all aspects of their planned care, including plans for breastfeeding. Male partners and other close family members are encouraged to attend the classes, which run for 2 h per week for 6 weeks. One evening is devoted to breastfeeding education, which is made fun by viewing videos and participating in group work. It is quite usual that the fathers-to-be attend; they are considered very important in the support and encouragement of their partners.

The curriculum for antenatal education includes preparation for breastfeeding, breast size, shape, and function, breastfeeding in hospital, breastfeeding at home, coping with conflicting or contradictory advice, support systems for enjoyable breastfeeding, common breastfeeding problems, the course of lactation, working and breastfeeding, and weaning.

Step Four, help mothers to initiate breastfeeding within half an hour of birth, has its own interpretation in Australia. More and more midwives and doctors are recognizing that it is important to keep the mother and baby together right from the moment of birth. The immediate skin-to-skin contact has the added advantage of keeping the baby warm. Many midwives have learned to rethink the order of their work and to make the first breastfeed a priority. It is being recognized increasingly that individual babies take varying amounts of time to seek the breast and start to breastfeed; the average is longer than the prescribed half-an-hour. The vital thing is that they have the opportunity, and that there is no interference or forcing.

Step Five is to show mothers how to breastfeed and how to maintain lactation even if they should be separated from their infants. The success of this step is very much dependent on the level of knowledge and skills of the midwives. As they are once again learning to teach mothers they need to be helped and supported themselves. We are at the stage at which the midwives are increasing their understanding of the process of breastfeeding and lactation, and taking the next step of being able to teach the mothers how to do this independently. Our midwives have had to become very skilled at hand-expressing breast milk. It is quite puzzling that so many babies do not learn early how to suckle effectively. We frequently need to take the remedial action of expressing and tea-spooning or cup feeding the breast milk to the baby, until the baby learns to breastfeed properly. Why does this happen? Is it the type of birth? Is it the analgesic or anaesthetic drugs used in labour? Is it connected with the artificial rupture of membranes? Is it the induced labour? Can it be traced back to the cramped position *in utero* or pre-birth thumb sucking? Is it connected with the new enthusiasm for placing the baby to the breast quickly after delivery – is it *too* quickly?

If the baby needs extra milk because of ineffective suckling, or if the mother and baby are necessarily separated because of illness or prematurity, it is now well-known that early milk removal is essential for long-term lactation. Most midwives know to start the expressing process as soon as possible and to continue this regularly (aiming for six to eight times per day). Back-up literature for the mother is very helpful –

preferably as concise as possible. The most important thing, however, is support and encouragement together with practical skills.

Step Six requires staff to give new-born infants of breastfeeding mothers no food or drink other than breast milk, unless medically indicated. Formerly, it had been common to give even healthy term babies extra water or formula 'just in case', without any regard to the implications. Over recent years the importance of exclusive breastfeeding to the immature infant's immune system has become better recognized. Also, our population has a high incidence of asthma and other allergic disease (NH&MRC, 1991). Many health workers believe that this sensitivity can be traced to early, complementary, artificial milk feeds, and so are very careful to avoid these. Apart from the obvious health risks, the effect on the mother's lactation is recognized as serious. The mothers need to have confidence in their bodies' ability to nourish their infants; what they learn in hospital, they will continue at home. We have found that we really need to be very strong in counteracting family pressure to 'just give the baby a bottle'. A carefully worded consent form, which the mother is asked to sign prior to any form of supplementation being given to the baby, is very powerful and educative.

Step Seven requires the practice of 'rooming-in', allowing mothers and infants to remain together 24 hours a day. The success of this step is very much dependent on the motivation of the midwives, the support of the doctors, and the care the mother is willing to take in making herself and her baby a priority. Our hospital is local to most mother's homes. Many come from large, noisy second-generation migrant families. The postnatal woman receives very little rest, as social interaction is seen to be very important. In the maternity ward, there is one two-bed shared room and the rest are large single rooms, which should be perfect to allow rooming-in and bedding-in.

The mothers also attract huge numbers of visitors and phone calls. It would be interesting to know just how many breastfeeds are staved off to accommodate the entertainment of visitors. Even very well-motivated midwives find it difficult to convince the mothers that they need to rest during the day to allow for the physiological night feeds. Of course, if the doctor or a midwife, trying to be 'helpful', arrives and recommends nursery care for the night the battle is lost. A mother who is feeling a bit depleted and who has not rested for many hours will jump at the chance of a night's sleep and will often not be in a fit state to weigh up the consequences. If the baby is cared for separately from the mother, we do try to compromise and be supportive by at least taking the baby in for breastfeeds. Only occasionally does the mother refuse this and request artificial feeds. Most midwives are now very well able to discuss this with the mother, to be non-judgmental, but to ensure informed consent. Strangely, colleagues in other larger hospitals with shared multi-bed accommodation report that this is much less of an issue in their work place and that rooming-in is very much the done thing.

Step Eight, to encourage breastfeeding on demand, is becoming much easier as the baby's physiology and expected feed pattern is better understood. Mothers can be helped to see that this very tiny, dependent infant with a small stomach cannot be expected to wait several hours for the next breastfeed, although there will be some naturally occurring long breaks, most often in the mornings. Midwives can use their powers of observation and show mothers that new-born babies follow an expected pattern, provided that the breastfeeds are very efficient. Mothers can be shown how an effective breastfeed should feel and how to assess a good intake by the change in the baby's sucking pattern from quick, to long strong with short pauses, to the dreamy phase when the pauses become longer until the baby releases its grasp. She can be taught to read her baby's cues for feeds. This will best equip her to be an expert in natural unrestricted feeds.

Step Nine is to give no artificial teats or dummies to breastfeeding infants. The detrimental effect of a baby sucking artificial objects makes clear logical sense if one understands the oral process necessary for breastfeeding.

Universal acceptance of this fact is not easy in the Australian culture. Because of the large amount of bottle-feeding during previous years many people are stuck in a mind-set that babies 'need' extra sucking on a dummy, and that the only manner in which expressed breast milk can be given is by bottle. Changing this attitude is a real challenge, and one which has not yet been met. The best possible way is probably by peer-group pressure as more and more people become converted. We have not yet won the battle of the bottle, but dummies are not encouraged and are not available within the hospital. It is quite frustrating to observe that the parents are very keen to give dummies. They almost seem to be considered as essential equipment. Perhaps it is a symptom of our average two-child-per-family culture; most young child-bearing couples have had little or no experience in handling small babies and have not learned other comfort measures.

Step Ten requires us to foster the establishment of breastfeeding support groups and refer mothers to them on discharge from hospital. We are very fortunate to have excellent NMAA groups in our region. They are willing to visit and speak to the mothers and to offer them solid support when at home. The maternal and child health nurses who follow up each woman also have their own mothering support groups.

Northpark has provided a service called CLARE. This is an acronym for the Centre for Lactation Assessment Resource and Education. The women are able to return to a hospital postnatal support group for discussion and breastfeeding revision when the baby is about 2 weeks old. If there are any problems that require more intensive care, a day assessment service is provided by a lactation consultant one day per week. This is open to any woman in the community. Three mothers and babies come into the unit for the day. A comprehensive history is taken, including details of the pregnancy and birth, and the early and prior breastfeeding history. The history is designed to be used as a way of educating the mothers about breastfeeding, so the questions start many lively discussions. The mothers tend to form a very close and friendly group on the day and seem to be quite surprised that they are not the only ones who have problems. The most important aspect of the clinic is the clinical assessment of a breastfeed. This is also very helpful to the other mothers watching, as part of the problem in our culture seems to be that our child-bearing women have not seen proper breastfeeding at close hand.

Once a feed has been observed, the mother is taught what she is trying to achieve and some ways to do so. Several breastfeeds are observed and she and the baby have the opportunity to practise with support and supervision. The mother is taught skills that may have been missed in her prior care, such as hand expressing. Before the end of the day a plan is made for each mother and written out for her to take back to show her maternal and child health nurse. This plan sets out the reason for presenting, the initial assessment of the problem, the management plan, and a progress report of what has occurred during the day. A report is also sent to the referring doctor.

We have also formed a Breastfeeding Link Group, established for health professionals and lay counsellors in the community. This group meets monthly as an informal peer-support group. It is valuable to discuss various aspects of care and for different people to know and understand each other's work. It is an opportunity to share new breastfeeding information, to provide study opportunities, and to let people know what seminars and courses are available currently. The group includes hospital midwives, antenatal educators, general practitioners, Royal District Nursing Service midwives, maternal and child health nurses, trainee and trained nursing mothers' counsellors, and paediatric nurses. We have all learned a lot from one another and have a better understanding of the individual roles.

These, then, are the lessons from Northpark Hospital's experience. Many maternity hospitals all over Australia are currently working towards the BFHI accreditation. It is, perhaps, harder for the larger units with many more staff to effect change, and to address the training and education necessary. It is important for us all to take full advantage of the things that the umbrella of the BFHI can do for us in providing the best possible conditions for breastfeeding mothers and babies. This may mean that we are taking it slowly, but although we have not moved as quickly as some other countries into the accreditation process, the BFHI is alive and well in Australia.

REFERENCES

Health Department of Victoria (1990) *Ministerial Review of Birthing Services in Victoria.* Health Department Victoria, Melbourne.

Morrow, M. and Barraclough, S. (1993) Breastfeeding and public policy in Australia: Limitations of a nutritional focus. *Health Promotions International*, **8**: 135–146.

Murray, S. (1993) *Northpark Breastfeeding Protocol.* Northpark Private Hospital, Greenhills Road, Bundoora 3083, Victoria, Australia.

NH&MRC (1991) *Food Allergies in Children.* National Health and Medical Research Council, Canberra ACT, Australia.

Victorian Breastfeeding Guidelines (1994) *Promoting Breastfeeding.* Department of Health and Community Services, Melbourne, Australia.

Walker, M. (1993) A fresh look at the risks of artificial infant feeding. *Journal of Human Lactation*, **9**(2): 97–107.

WHO/UNICEF (1981) *International Code of Marketing of Breast-milk Substitutes.* World Health Organization, Geneva.

WHO/UNICEF (1989) *Protecting, Promoting and Supporting Breastfeeding: The Special Role of Maternity Services.* World Health Organization, Geneva.

CHAPTER

4

A Case Study from Myanmar: The Baby Friendly Home Delivery Project

Daw Mya Mya and **San San Myint**

Myanmar (previously known as Burma) is a country in South-East Asia, bordered by Thailand, Laos, and China in the east and by India and Bangladesh in the west. It has a population of 43 million, with 76% living in the rural areas. This case study describes how a pilot project adapted the concept of 'baby friendliness' to meet the particular situation of a rural population who give birth at home.

In 1971, Oo and Naing's study found that 95% of rural mothers were breastfeeding their infants up to the age of 12 months, and at 24–36 months, 30% of children were still receiving breast milk. Over 20 years later breastfeeding is still very much considered a natural process in the country. The majority of expectant mothers accept that they need to breastfeed their babies. Breastfeeding in public is a common practice in rural Myanmar and no one takes offence. However, what has become clear in recent years is that in spite of this continued acceptance of the centrality of breastfeeding, there are some problems with infant feeding practices.

The 1982–1983 Weaning Practices Survey (Nutrition Division, 1983) suggested that the initiation of breastfeeding often did not occur within 24 hours of delivery. Rates of initiation of breastfeeding on the first day of life in the country's different regions ranged from 11% to 43%. Furthermore, the introduction of complementary food before 3 months of age was found to occur in 13–50% of babies.

A recent study in a peri-urban area of Yangon Division indicated that 99.09% of mothers breastfed their infants (Oo, 1993). Nevertheless, only 4.5% of babies were exclusively breastfed by the age of 5 months. Complementary feeding was started as early as 1 month. By the age of 3 months, 66.8% of infants were receiving complementary food. It was also found that only 68% of mothers fed their babies on the day of birth.

One of the Myanmar health goals for children and women in the 1990s is to enable all women to breastfeed exclusively for 4–6 months, and to continue breastfeeding, with complementary food, well into the second year (National Programme of Action, 1993).

The Ministry of Health recognizes the significant benefits of breastfeeding and that a lack of 'optimal' feeding practices is endangering infant health. (Optimal feeding includes putting the baby to the breast as soon as possible after birth, giving of colostrum, breastfeeding on demand, exclusively breastfeeding until 4–6 months of age, and giving appropriate complementary food.)

In January 1993 Myanmar joined the UNICEF/WHO Baby Friendly Hospital Initiative (BFHI) to promote optimal breastfeeding in maternity facilities. The most recent scientific findings are now being used to promote and facilitate optimal breastfeeding practices in hospitals around the country. In Myanmar, 58 hospitals have already received the BFHI Achievement Award.

However, as over 80% of babies are born at home in Myanmar, it seemed important to promote breastfeeding beyond the hospitals, so the Baby Friendly Home Delivery (BFHD) project was conceived. An innovative approach had to be devised to reach the rural community. Mothers delivering in non-urban areas are attended by the midwives (60%), auxiliary midwives (AMWs, 10–20%), or traditional birth attendants (TBAs, 5–10%) (Ministry of Health 1993). In order to reach the rural mothers and encourage systematic breastfeeding, the attendants involved in domiciliary delivery would have to be trained in baby friendly practice.

THE PROJECT

The goal of the pilot project was to identify strategies for providing optimal feeding to all babies delivered at home in one township, and then apply the successful strategies to all townships throughout the country.

Hlegu (*Figure 4.1*) was chosen for the pilot study. It lies 25 miles north of Yangon City, the capital of Myanmar. It has been the study area for many health projects and the health infrastructure is more compact than in other rural townships in the country. Baseline data collection was performed in January 1994.

The township has a 50-bed hospital with 10 doctors and 10 nurses, two smaller station hospitals, an MCH Centre, a Rural Health Centre, and a Rural Health Subcentre which supervises 73 AMWs and 173 TBAs (*Figure 4.2*).

Figure 4.1 Hlegu township.

Population	146,343
Size	1495.5 km^2
Population density/ km^2	98
Houses	
urban	3425
rural	25,179
total	28,604

Attendant/Hospital	Births
Midwives	2161
Auxiliary midwives	300
TBAs	309
Township Hospital	214
Station Hospital (1)	58
Station Hospital (2)	45

Figure 4.2 Attendants at deliveries in 1993 (total births, 3087).

There are five important steps in the development and establishment of a functioning BFHD programme: establish the key messages, formulate a training plan and train the trainers, who had to train all home birth attendants (the midwives, AMWs, and trained TBAs), who would in turn give the mothers the knowledge needed for successful breastfeeding and optimal infant feeding practices. The fifth and final step is to evaluate the BFHD.

THE MESSAGES – OUR 'TEN STEPS'

The messages were based on the *Ten Steps to Successful Breastfeeding* (UNICEF/WHO, 1989) – see Chapter 1, Appendix II, page 19 – with a few alterations tailored to the needs of the rural community. These ten steps (see box on page 50) address several existing and potential problems of breastfeeding for infants born at home in Myanmar. In Step One, we substituted a national policy for the hospital breastfeeding policy. Steps Two through to Six are the same as in the BFHI. Step Seven of the BFHI was omitted, because in home deliveries mothers and babies invariably sleep in one room or in one bed. Steps Eight and Nine of the BFHI thus become Steps Seven and Eight of the BFHD. In Step Nine of the BFHD, breastfeeding support groups should be established and minor problems of breastfeeding recognized, managed, or referred. Step Ten was added because the custom in Myanmar is to use rice as the sole complementary food between 0–6 months (Myint, 1987; Win, 1993) and most mothers are reluctant to feed their babies animal protein and vegetables. This results in under-nutrition among infants and toddlers, so babies tend to fall off the weight-for-age centile after the introduction of complementary foods. For this reason, knowledge and practice as to the proper choice of complementary food has been emphasized, although it does not feature in the original 'ten steps'.

Ten Steps to Successful Breastfeeding Home Delivery (BFHD)

1. Have a written national breastfeeding policy that is routinely communicated to all health care staff.
2. Train all health care staff in the skills necessary to implement this policy.
3. Inform all pregnant women about the benefits and management of breastfeeding.
4. Help mothers initiate breastfeeding within half-an-hour of birth.
5. Show mothers how to breastfeed, and how to maintain lactation even if they should be separated from the infant.
6. Give the new-born infant no food or drink other than breast milk until 4–6 months old.
7. Encourage breastfeeding on demand.
8. Give no artificial teats or pacifiers to breastfeeding infants.
9. Foster the establishment of breastfeeding support groups and make mothers know where to seek help in the face of problems in breastfeeding.
10. Encourage mothers to continue breastfeeding their children until the age of 2 years and help them choose appropriate complementary foods.

These ten steps then formed the basis for ten specific tasks that needed to be carried out by home birth attendants (see box on page 51). To convey the messages, learning materials were developed. A text was written to give appropriate and adequate explanations as to the benefits of breastfeeding, its management, problems in feeding, and appropriate weaning practices. A booklet was also produced with a pictorial display of each of the ten tasks. This was developed by a group of specialists interested in lactation management, and was primarily aimed at the TBAs, most of whom have less than primary level education. A complementary feeding schedule was suggested, as shown in *Figure 4.3*.

Month	Food
5	rice + oil
5–6	rice (4) + lentil/meat/fish (1) + oil
6–9	rice (4) + lentil/meat/fish (1) + vegetable (1) + oil rice (4) + meat/fish (1) + lentil (1) + vegetable (1) + oil

Always add oil; feed baby 2 hourly; give fruits.

Figure 4.3 Complementary feeding schedule.

Tasks for Home Birth Attendants

- Task 1. To be familiar with the national breastfeeding policy.
- Task 2. To be trained for BFHD.
- Task 3. To give antenatal health education on breastfeeding, including the benefits of breastfeeding, an understanding of a balanced diet, the daily nutritional requirements of a pregnant mother, personal hygiene and preparation of the nipples, and – breastfeeding technique – for example, that the areola should be included during suckling.
- Task 4. To assist mothers to put the baby to the breast immediately after delivery, after giving the initial immediate care to the new-born (drying the baby and not bathing it).
- Task 5. To assist effective breastfeeding by aiding in proper positioning and attachment of the baby for breastfeeding, and by showing how to detach the baby from the breast, how to sustain lactation, and how to express breast milk. In cases of separation from the mother, to teach how to feed expressed breast milk with a spoon or cup.
- Task 6. To teach mothers to breastfeed exclusively for the first 4 months, giving no breast milk substitutes, no water, no honey, no gruel, and no rice.
- Task 7. To teach mothers to feed babies on demand, avoiding rigid clock feeding.
- Task 8. To inform mothers not to give pacifiers or artificial teats.
- Task 9. (a) To establish breastfeeding support groups; and (b) To identify and solve simple problems during breastfeeding or refer those who require more specialized attention. Attendants should be able to recognize and act appropriately upon maternal problems, such as cracked nipples, breast engorgement, blocked ducts, mastitis, and breast abscess. They should also be able to advise on the feeding of twins and to identify infant problems, such as low birth weight, malformations, and jaundice.
- Task 10. To encourage the continuation of breastfeeding up to the age of 2 years and the introduction of complementary food only after at least 4 months.

TRAINING

The midwives and others assisting home delivery are the key actors for the BFHD. For a township to become completely 'Baby Friendly', not only would all the hospitals have to meet the criteria of BFHI, but also all midwives and others assisting home delivery would need to have the knowledge and skills to apply effectively at least eight out of the ten steps. It is necessary, therefore, to provide them with new knowledge and additional skills through training.

The first training in BFHI was that of the future trainers. These included the Township Medical Officer, one Hospital Medical Officer, one School Health Medical Officer, and one Lady Health Visitor, who were trained by a team of breastfeeding specialists in Yangon City. They then served as a core group to educate the health staff of Hlegu Township in breastfeeding, conducting courses for doctors, nurses, health assistants, lady health visitors, and midwives who were in government service. These trainees then trained 52 midwives, 73 AMWs, and 79 trained TBAs, with the aid of the printed materials already mentioned. A video tape demonstrating the ten steps of the BFHD was also used. The AMWs and TBAs received a minimum of 18 h training, including 3 h of practical work. Extra time was given to the TBAs. An interactive type of training was utilized for these adult learners.

Besides the home birth attendants, 66 volunteers from Myanmar Maternal and Child Welfare Association (MMCWA) also attended the training course. The MMCWA is a non-governmental organization involved in working with mothers and children. They were trained with the aim of forming a network of breastfeeding support groups.

The plan is that those mothers who attend the antenatal clinics are given health education on the benefits and management of breastfeeding. For those who cannot attend the clinic, the midwife, AMW, or TBA will educate them, either alone or in small groups in their homes. The dissemination of this breastfeeding knowledge will be enhanced by the use and distribution of pamphlets, audio visual aids, or models or charts during health education.

EVALUATION OF THE BABY FRIENDLY HOME DELIVERY PROJECT

The evaluation of BFHD was planned at the time that the text and handbook were drafted, reviewed, and field-tested. The evaluation procedures were based on the BFHI assessment format. First, there is a self-assessment questionnaire to be utilized once the training is over and implementation of the project has been satisfactory. Then the Township Health Authority will invite in the Regional Assessment Team, and the results will be utilized for further improvements in the programme.

REFERENCES

Ministry of Health (1993) *Country Health Profile, Myanmar, April 1993.* Department of Planning and Statistics, Ministry of Health, Yangon.

Myint, Y.S. (1987) *A study on Child Rearing Practices in Urban and Rural Areas.* Dissertation submitted for Master of Medical Science in Paediatrics.

National Programme of Action (1993) *Myanmar Goals for Women and Children in the 1990.*

Nutrition Division (1983) *Weaning Practices Survey 1982–1983.* Department of Health.

Oo, T.T. (1978) *Supplementary Feeding Practices at Htaukkyant Village.* A Study from the Department of Medical Research.

Oo, T.T. and Naing, K.M. (1985) Breastfeeding and weaning practices for infants and young children. *Food and Nutrition Bulletin,* 7: 47–52.

Oo, Y.Y. (1993) *Infant Feeding and Weaning Practices in a Peri-Urban Area of Yangon Division.* Dissertation submitted for Master of Medical Sciences in Paediatrics.

UNICEF/WHO (1989) *Protecting, Promoting, and Supporting Breastfeeding: The Special Role of Maternity Services.* The World Health Organization, Geneva.

Win, T. (1993) *Child Rearing Practices and Social Class in Urban and Rural Yangon Division.* Dissertation submitted for Master of Medical Science in Paediatrics.

CHAPTER 5

A Case Study from Namibia: The National Mother Baby Friendly Initiative

Esther H. Viljoen and **Justina N. Amadhila**

Breastfeeding provides the optimal method for feeding infants, especially in the first 6 months of life, during which no other foods are necessary for growth. Breastfeeding is more than just a way of feeding a baby, it promotes bonding and love between the mother and her child, and contributes enormously to its early development. It was with this in mind that the Baby and Mother Friendly Initiative (BMFI) was launched by Dr Sam Nujoma, His Excellency the President of Namibia, on 9 October 1992, at a public rally in Windhoek (Nujoma, 1992):

> *Today we are starting a new consciousness in Namibia and I am calling upon all members of our communities to start a movement which will help us to care for women and children who are among the most vulnerable in our society.*

This was the Namibian response to the global initiative known as Baby Friendly Hospital Initiative (BFHI), which focuses on the promotion of breastfeeding and elimination of the use of breast-milk substitutes in hospitals; in Namibia, this initiative was to be broadened to include support for mothers and children in all health facilities, in the home environment, and at work places.

BREASTFEEDING IN NAMIBIA

In spite of the many advantages of breastfeeding, there has been an apparent decline in breastfeeding among the younger generation of women, especially in the urban areas. Studies conducted in Katutura (Windhoek) and two small towns in the south, found 54% of mothers with 3-month-old babies were breastfeeding, dropping to 15% for those with 12-month-old babies (Hughson, 1986).

The Household Health and Nutrition Survey conducted among 300 children under the age of 2 years in the peri-urban areas of Oshakati and Ondangwa in the North West Region (NISSER, 1991) found that 97% of these children aged 0–6 months were being breastfed, dropping to 50% of the 13–18-month-olds, and to 20% of those aged 19 months and above (MOHSS/UNICEF, 1990). The Namibian Demographic Health Survey indicates that 97% of women do initiate breastfeeding. However, many mothers stop breastfeeding after 4 months, because they go back to work (DHS, 1992).

It is evident that in Namibia, in both urban and rural areas, solids are often introduced too early (at 2 months) or too late (9 months). In the rural areas, breastfeeding practices may be affected by women's heavy work-loads. There are many matriarchal households – only 42% of women aged 15–49 years are in a matrimonial union (DHS, 1992) – and the trend in urban areas in Namibia has been towards an increasing number of working mothers. Women have to return to work within 1–3 months after delivery, because shortcomings in the Labour Act mean that the 3 months' maternity leave is unpaid. Employers have often been reluctant to allow mothers access to their babies to maintain lactation, and in the majority of instances breastfeeding facilities were non-existent (MOHSS, 1992).

Births in institutions account for 85% of those in urban areas and 58% of those in rural areas (DHS, 1992). Before the implementation of the BMFI, it was believed that a baby must have its own bed, and most maternity hospitals in Namibia were equipped with baby cots. Babies were also taken to the nursery during visiting time. In some facilities the mothers had insufficient contact with their babies. This inhibited their milk supply, and resulted in unrealistic expectations of their baby's behaviour because they had so little involvement in its initial care. In hospital, they were also exposed to the idea that the milk would only 'come in' on the third day, and that the baby would need infant formula until then. Newcomers to the city came to believe that this was the correct way to do things. Formula was distributed at feeding time, and at discharge. Feedings were scheduled according to hospital routines, and not according to the baby's needs. Health personnel were untrained in how to help women maintain a milk supply when separated from their infants. In many ways hospitals and their routines were one of the main obstacles to exclusive breastfeeding.

There was much advertising of infant formula, bottles, and teats alongside images of beautiful babies in television programmes, newspapers, supermarkets, and chemists shops. The mother from the rural area began to view an attractive bottle and teat as both modern and prestigious, while breastfeeding was outmoded. Even among well-educated and discerning urban mothers, the seeds of uncertainty and doubt were sown.

THE BABY AND MOTHER FRIENDLY INITIATIVE IN NAMIBIA: ONE COUNTRY'S VISION

The BMFI in Namibia is adapted from the global BFHI aimed at protecting, promoting, and supporting breastfeeding in hospitals. In Namibia, the scope of the initiative has been extended in several ways. It includes the mother because the baby cannot be seen in isolation; the needs of the mother need to be taken into account to enable her to take effective care of her baby. The hospital environment is no longer referred to specifically, because the initiative also aims to promote breastfeeding in work places and in homes. Lastly, the initiative aims also to promote other interventions, including immunization, family planning, and good nutrition for mothers and children.

Community participation plays an important role. Mothers need to be well-informed for them to be able to choose what suits them best. Mothers should not be forced to breastfeed by health workers, but rather it should be the women themselves who insist on breastfeeding their babies. They should also demand that their right to breastfeed, and their babies' right to be breastfed, is respected by employers.

The overall objective of the BMFI is to contribute to the survival, development, and protection of the child as well as to improve the health status of mothers. It is seen as integral to the country's broader goals for children and women in the 1990s:

- Between 1990 and 2000 to reduce infant and under 5-year-old mortality by one-third to 50/1000 and 70/1000 live births, respectively (figures based on DHS, 1992).
- To reduce maternal mortality rate (MMR) to 50% of the 1990 levels –MMR is currently estimated at 225/100,000 live births (DHS, 1992).
- To reduce severe and moderate malnutrition among under 5-year-olds to 50% of 1990 levels. (According to the DHS (1992), 9% were severely malnourished and 28% suffered moderate malnutrition.)

As already stated, BMFI was launched on 9th October 1992 by His Excellency, Dr Sam Nujoma, the President of the Republic of Namibia. Furthermore, the Minister of Health and Social Services issued a Breastfeeding Policy based on the global *Ten Steps to Successful Breastfeeding* (see Chapter 1, Appendix II, page 19). While awaiting the adoption of the National Code for Marketing of Breast-milk Substitutes, a Ministerial Directive was issued stating that no free or low-cost breast-milk substitutes should be distributed to health facilities.

The BMFI has some specific objective targets (Government of Namibia/UNICEF, 1991):

- 80% of all health facilities in Namibia will be baby and mother friendly by 1997 according to the agreed criteria.
- 75% of all mothers will practise exclusive breastfeeding for the first 4–6 months by the end of 1997.
- At least 25% of work places will have baby and mother friendly corners by the end of 1997.
- There will be increased access to other preventive and promotive interventions for children and mothers, such as good nutrition, immunization, correct treatment for diarrhoea, and family spacing.
- The adoption of a National Code of Marketing of Breast-milk Substitutes, based on the International Code of Breast-milk Substitutes, by the end of 1995.

In most countries, BFHI has focused on the promotion of the Ten Steps to Successful Breastfeeding in hospitals, especially in maternity units. In Namibia it has also provided the opportunity for consolidating child survival, establishing development and protection initiatives, and promoting the health status of mothers.

The initiative in Namibia aims to create a friendly environment for child and mother from birth, with an initial focus on good nutrition for both of them. Breastfeeding which starts immediately after birth has numerous advantages, and it is considered the responsibility of all who interact with the mother and child to ensure its successful introduction and sustainability for at least 2 years, with an appropriate and timely introduction of complementary feeding after 4–6 months.

In order to promote breastfeeding there must be a suitable environment for mother and baby at birth. Attention is therefore paid in the BMFI guidelines (MOHSS, 1992), to the attitudes of the personnel towards their patients, to whether fathers or other members of the family are allowed to attend and support mothers in labour, and to whether the mothers are allowed to give birth in the position of their choice. Focusing on the need for the family, and especially the father, to be supportive at the stage of labour and delivery is a key issue. Fathers have not always been supportive. The obligation of staff to provide and maintain a calm and supportive atmosphere in the labour ward is also emphasized.

THE CHALLENGE

In order to move towards becoming a BMFI Nation, factors which negatively influence breastfeeding need to be addressed. The initiative must (MOHSS, 1992):

- Enable the child to receive the natural protection and nutrition of breastfeeding.
- Promote the role of fathers, families, and communities.
- Enable health workers, employers, leaders, and planners to develop new and positive attitudes towards mothers and children.
- Ensure that there is a reduction of the mother's work-load, to enable her to nurture her baby, by obtaining the father's support.
- Provide access to immunization of children and women.
- Provide access to treatment of common diseases, such as acute respiratory infections and diarrhoea.
- Ensure that family spacing methods are offered.
- Facilitate good nutrition being offered to mothers and children.
- Ensure an increased allocation of resources to programmes that have an impact on the health and welfare of children and women.
- Promote the fight against women and child abuse, and alcohol and drug abuse.

Through this initiative Namibia will have affirmed the right of every child, as well as its mother, to be nourished adequately and to be protected from disease.

THE STRATEGIES

The following strategies were specified for the implementation of the BMFI (MOHSS, 1992):

- Broadening the approach to include all health facilities, work places, and home environments.
- Training of health workers on various aspects concerning breastfeeding, focusing on the Ten Steps to Successful Breastfeeding, and to improve their attitudes towards mothers and children.
- Adoption of an inter-sectoral approach in the creation of a friendly environment for mother and baby, including working together with breastfeeding support groups.
- Advocacy for increased paid maternity leave for working mothers.
- Creation of baby friendly corners in work places.

- Advocacy for the BMFI among all civil leaders, policymakers, planners, and religious leaders.
- Education of the public in general on the key areas addressed by the initiative through social mobilization strategies.
- Encouragement of networking among groups and agencies, including breast-feeding support groups.
- Recognition and promotion of the role of fathers in supporting the breastfeeding mother.
- Integration of the initiative into other primary health care (PHC) activities, such as nutrition, safe motherhood, and control of diarrhoeal diseases and immunization.
- Promotion of good nutrition for the pregnant and lactating mother.

It was recommended during the national Safe Motherhood conference, held in Windhoek in November 1991 (MOHSS, 1991), that Namibia should draw up guidelines in order to implement these strategies. It was also recognized that the first step towards reaching the aims of BMFI would need to be a positive change in health personnel's attitudes. The promotion of the Ten Steps to Successful Breastfeeding therefore became an essential means to prepare for the wider BMFI.

THE TASK FORCE

A national task force for the planning, implementation, monitoring, and evaluation of the BMFI was formed with members from non-governmental organizations, the Breast-Feeding Association of Namibia, La Leche League of Namibia, the Ministry of Health and Social Services, Department of Women's Affairs, the Ministry of Regional and Local Government and Housing, the Ministry of Information and Broadcasting, the Ministry of Youth and Sport, UNICEF, WHO, UNFPA (United Nations Fund for Population Activities), and women's groups.

Terms of reference for the National Task Force were:

1. To co-ordinate BMFI activities.
2. To review the material available on BMFI, especially the International Code of Marketing of Breast Milk Substitutes.
3. To develop a National Code of Marketing of Breast-milk Substitutes.
4. To mobilize communities towards being baby and mother friendly.
5. To conduct supervisory visits to the regions.
6. To conduct internal and external assessment for baby and mother friendly facilities.
7. To give technical support in baby and mother friendly training in the regions.
8. To create awareness among employees and employers of government sectors, private sectors, and non-governmental organizations to establish baby and mother friendly areas at work places.
9. To develop material for breastfeeding training.
10. To supply information material specifically for support groups for breastfeeding.
11. To develop supportive measures for mothers, e.g. maternity leave and flexitime.
12. To assess the progress made and to write reports on BMFI activities.
13. To disseminate information and share experiences through the Ministry of Health and Social Services by publishing articles quarterly in the newsletter *PHC in Action*.

THE TEN STEPS AS A FIRST PHASE

The World Health Organization (WHO) and UNICEF recommended that the criteria for declaring a health facility 'Baby Friendly' should be based on the Ten Steps to Successful Breastfeeding. These global criteria have been modified to suit the Namibian situation. All health facilities in Namibia have a major role to play in implementing BMFI. In order to reach effectively the families, BMFI has to reach not only the hospitals, but also all community-based health care facilities; it has to change attitudes towards mothers and babies who visit clinics, eliminate the distribution of free and low-cost breast-milk substitutes in hospitals and clinics, and ensure that adequate health education, focusing on promotion of breast milk, is provided.

Such a comprehensive change requires in-service courses in health facilities for all categories of medical workers and traditional birth attendants (TBAs). The first National Training of Trainers was held in June 1993. The trainer's task is to conduct the training of all health workers in their various health facilities, and to foster the establishment of support groups to which mothers can be referred to on discharge from hospital. The following steps were suggested in order to certify a health facility as 'BMFI approved':

- Awareness should be created among all staff of that specific health facility.
- Each health facility then declares its intention to be baby and mother friendly according to the established criteria.
- The Division of Family and Community Health and the National Task Force provide training materials, videos on the BMFI Policy Statement, and BMFI Guidelines and posters on BMFI.
- The health facility strategically displays the BMFI policy statement, and ensures that all staff members are aware of it. There should be no display or promoting of any marketing material for breast-milk substitutes.
- The health facility should examine the Global Criteria, assess its needs and practices accordingly, and arrange for the collection of baseline information.
- Further, the health facility should be able to demonstrate an outline of its health education programme, indicating how many hours of training were received by mothers and health personnel. Adequate training of staff, according to training guidelines developed by the National Task Force, should be conducted. The training should therefore be at least 18 h in total, including a minimum of 3 h of supervised clinical experience, and cover at least eight of the Ten Steps to Successful Breastfeeding.
- The health facility should conduct a self-appraisal, using the Request for Assessment Form and the Self-Appraisal Form provided by the BMFI Task Force.
- The facility should than invite, through the PHC Director, the National Assessors within the BMFI to conduct an assessment of the facility.
- The National Task Force then informs the facility as to when the internal assessment will be conducted.
- Following the internal assessment, the Task Force will recommend the facility for external assessment.

The criteria used for qualifying the hospitals is an 80% score for BMFI achievement and 70% score for commitment, based on the Ten Steps to Successful Breastfeeding.

The National Task Force invites external assessors from other countries and from UNICEF, IBFAN (International Baby Food Action Network), and WHO to evaluate the progress made in Namibia. Of 36 hospitals, 17 have so far been declared baby and mother friendly by external assessors.

BABY FRIENDLY CORNERS

One important element of the BMFI is to establish baby friendly corners. These provide facilities for a lactating, working mother to express breast milk and store it for her baby at home. They enable a working mother to feed the baby when the child minder is able to bring him or her in for a feed during the day. They further enable a working mother whose child minder is occasionally absent to come to work with her infant 'just for the day', and thus to reduce absenteeism. They make it possible for lactating mothers who attend meetings, seminars, and conferences to be with their children and in a friendly environment. The corners can also serve to facilitate the dissemination of information on various child survival interventions, including immunization and oral rehydration solution.

A baby friendly corner does not have the same status as a crèche, where children are left by the parent to be cared for by others. It is better viewed as an extension of the home environment. The working mother, as well as co-workers, have to participate actively in the creation of a baby friendly corner. Similarly, those who organize meetings should ensure that there is a room or place designed as a 'corner for the mother', where she can breastfeed her child. Employers have an important role to play to ensure that baby friendly corners are established as a welfare measure to support the lactating mother.

Basic requirements for the baby friendly corner are:

- Adequate toilet facilities.
- A table on which to change the child's nappies.
- A chair for the mother to rest on while she is breastfeeding, or while expressing breast milk for the child who is at home or in a crèche.
- A cot for the infant.
- A wash basin or sink (for hand washing).
- Where possible, there should be a fridge for storing expressed breast milk, and complementary feeds for the older infant.

The criteria for declaring a work place BMFI approved are currently being further developed and agreed upon in consultation with employers and employees, both in the private sector and in government.

THE BMFI IN THE HOME ENVIRONMENT

The involvement and participation of the other family and household members in the support of breastfeeding cannot be overemphasized. Fathers and older children need to be sensitized to support breastfeeding, along with other child survival interventions, such as immunization, nutrition, the correct management of diarrhoea and acute respiratory infections, family planning, and sanitation. This can be done by dissemination of information packages at household level. Furthermore, division of labour among members of the family needs to be encouraged, to reduce the mother's work-load. Fathers in particular need to become more supportive, taking more responsibility for family care.

THE FUTURE

The success of the initiative depends largely on the extent to which community participation and involvement is achieved. The political will and support for this exists, but needs to be maintained. The preparation and dissemination of relevant breastfeeding information packages to target groups, such as community leaders, families, youth groups, women groups, hospitals, clinics, created breastfeeding corners, and religious leaders is an ongoing activity.

The formulation of breastfeeding support groups, especially at the community level, is in its infancy stage, but will be promoted. Groups, such as women's groups, TBAs, The Breastfeeding Association, and community health workers will need to be mobilized to support this initiative. The Global Breastfeeding Week will be celebrated yearly, supported by national radio and television.

In order to achieve the objectives of BMFI, adequate resources need to be mobilized within the context of on-going programmes. The BMFI in Namibia has largely been supported by UNICEF, with other funding mobilized by WHO and UNFPA.

ACKNOWLEDGEMENTS

Finally, we wish to acknowledge the contribution of Mrs Ella Shihepo, Head of Nutrition, and the technical support from Dr Orinda, UNICEF Health Project Officer, in the development of BMFI Guidelines in Namibia.

REFERENCES

DHS (Demographic Health Survey) (1992) *Namibia Demographic Health Survey.* Macro International Inc., Columbia, pp 114–118.

Hughson, H. (1986), *Survey of National Status and Related Factors in Selected Areas of Namibia.* Report prepared for OXFAM.

Government of Namibia/UNICEF (1991) Country programme of co-operation. In: *Programme Plans of Operation 1992–1996.* Government of Namibia/UNICEF, Windhoek, pp 44–47.

MOHSS (1991a) *Proceedings of the National Safe Motherhood Conference, 26–28 November, Windhoek.* Ministry of Health and Social Services, Windhoek. Unpublished document, pp 66–71.

MOHSS (1991b) *National Programme of Action for the Children in Namibia.* Ministry of Health and Social Services, Windhoek.

MOHSS (1992) Towards a baby and mother friendly nation. In: *The Baby and Mother Friendly Initiative Guidelines.* Ministry of Health and Social Services, Windhoek.

MOHSS/UNICEF (1990) *Household Health and Nutrition in Namibia: Report on a Survey in Katutura.* Ministry of Health and Social Services, Windhoek. Unpublished document.

NISSER (1991) *Situation Analysis of Children and Women in Namibia.* Ministry of Health and Social Services, Windhoek.

Nujoma, S. (1992) *Speech by the President of the Republic of Namibia to Launch the BMFI,* 9 October 1992, Windhoek. Unpublished material.

The Commercial Pressures against Baby Friendliness

Patti Rundall

INTRODUCTION

The adoption of the *International Code of Marketing of Breast-milk Substitutes*, hereafter '*The Code*', in 1981 was an acknowledgement by the world – including the baby food industry – that aggressive marketing of breast-milk substitutes was posing a serious threat to the well-being of infants everywhere (WHO, 1981). At that time the World Health Organization (WHO) estimated that 1.5 million infants died each year because they were not breastfed. The number of infants who suffered episodes of illness that could be prevented by exclusive breastfeeding far exceeded this number. *The Code* was an important breakthrough in consumer protection which could, if properly used, make a significant contribution to infant health and well-being. However, 15 years later, these figures have not reduced.

In this chapter I examine how *The Code* was developed, and the way that the baby food industry has responded to the pressure to change its marketing methods – its ability to absorb and minimize *The Code*'s provisions and its remarkable skill in manipulating *The Code* to its own advantage. Finally, I outline some of the things that need to be done to make *The Code* effective.

THE NEED FOR AN INTERNATIONAL CODE OF MARKETING

Breast-milk substitutes (infant formula, bottle-fed weaning foods, etc.) compete with a product that is not on sale. Breast milk does not have the benefit of being 'marketed', it is never packaged or labelled, nor is it promoted in glossy brochures and magazines with the same intensity as its substitutes. This has caused an imbalance in the information and advice that mothers and carers receive. In recognition of this, the *International Code of Marketing of Breast-milk Substitutes* was devised. It aimed to remove commercial pressures from the arena of infant feeding so as to ensure that all mothers could be given accurate, impartial advice. There had been a world-wide decline in breastfeeding, and as *The Code*'s preamble stated (WHO, 1981):

> ... *in view of the vulnerability of infants in the early months of life and the risks involved in inappropriate feeding practices ... the marketing of breast-milk substitutes requires special treatment.*

The Code arose out of a struggle in which the conflicting interests of health and profit were brought to the fore. Governments, United Nations agencies, non-governmental organizations (NGOs) representing consumers and health professionals, and the infant food manufacturers (including some of the world's largest food and pharmaceutical transnational companies) were all involved.

Despite their fierce opposition to *The Code* prior to its adoption, the baby food companies' official public position since 1981 has been one of support for *The Code*; indeed, by 1984 some companies were even claiming to be its leading proponents. An editorial in *Nestlé News* (Nestlé, 1984) claimed:

> *Nestlé was one of the main parties recommending the creation of a code, for without a code our practices would be forever steeped in controversy .... Nestlé views the situation today as one that has evolved naturally .... To us, this has been a continuity of trying our level best to implement The Code and to actually hammer out exactly what The Code calls for.*

The real history and continuity of action, however, was very different. Socio-economic changes, the changing roles of women in society, and the internationalization of trade are acknowledged to be important factors which have affected infant-feeding practices. However, the problem is also closely linked with health-worker attitudes to childbirth and infant feeding. These underwent radical changes during the nineteenth and early part of the twentieth century in Europe and the United States, as the medical profession attempted to take control. Ignorant of the physiology of breastfeeding, they interfered with that process – they separated mothers and babies, limited feed times, and unwittingly turned breastfeeding into a 'problem' for many women. Lactation failure was soon accepted as normal and artificial feeding as the solution.

The medical profession thus, albeit unintentionally, played an important role in the creation and expansion of the baby food market. The baby food companies took full commercial advantage of the situation and promoted their products in developed and developing countries alike. Some outstanding doctors tried to draw the world's attention to the malnutrition and disease which resulted.

One such critic was Dr Cicely Williams, the paediatrician well-known for her work on kwashiorkor. As early as 1939 she condemned publicly the spread of artificial feeding and the promotion tactics used by the companies. In a lecture to the Singapore Rotary Club entitled 'Milk and Murder' she stated (Williams, 1939):

> *If you are legal purists you may wish me to change the title of this address to 'Milk and Manslaughter'. But if your lives were as embittered as mine is, by seeing day after day this massacre of the innocents by unsuitable feeding, then I believe you would feel as I do that misguided propaganda on infant feeding should be punished as the most criminal form of sedition, and that these deaths should be regarded as murder.*

Nearly 40 years on she was still speaking out, and scathingly commenting on the industry's use of what it called 'milk nurses' (Williams, 1978):

> *I went to Singapore and found Nestlé nurses, these girls dressed as nurses, dragging a good lactating breast out of a baby's mouth and pouring in baby milks.*

By the 1960s, concerned doctors had started to draw attention to the radio adverts which were being broadcast regularly in Africa (SAFEP, 1975):

> *Mother, believe in Lactogen .... All the things in mother's milk are also present in Lactogen. Mother watch the health of your baby, and give him the best, give Lactogen.*

The evidence which linked malnutrition with artificial feeding had grown in the years following World War II, and by 1968 Dr Derrick Jelliffe, Director of the Caribbean Food and Nutrition Institute in Jamaica, was describing the conditions caused by artificial feeding as 'commerciogenic malnutrition' (Jelliffe, 1971). He called for a dialogue between health professionals and the infant food industry to resolve the problem. During the 1970s Dr Jelliffe and other paediatricians organized a series of meetings with the baby food industry, and agencies such as UNICEF and the Food and Agriculture Organization (FAO). There was disagreement over the extent of the problem, but consensus was reached with the 1972 Protein–Calorie Advisory Group (PAG) Statement No. 23, which stated (PAG, 1972):

> *... that promotion [of infant formula] to mothers in hospital was inappropriate*

and called for an end to promotion that might discourage breastfeeding. However the statement failed to address some of the fundamental problems, and almost appeared to endorse sales of breast-milk substitutes rather than protect breastfeeding, by suggesting that:

> *In any country lacking breast-milk substitutes, it is urgent that infant formulas be developed and introduced .... Governments should ... provide also for free distribution of these foods to the vulnerable groups in the lowest income families ... encourage recognition of promotion as an essential component of any marketing programme to establish widespread consumer use of nutritious foods for children.*

What had started as an important health initiative had somehow been transformed into a public relations victory for the baby food industry, which now had the official stamp of UN approval. Indeed, this process demonstrated to the companies the advantages of discussion and collaboration with the UN and with health workers. Were it not for the involvement of the NGOs, the industry's expansion strategy would then have continued unimpeded.

During the 1970s, pressure for change in baby food markets mounted. Opposition groups became more and more organized and many articles, films, and books on the issue were published. Two law suits, in particular, received considerable media attention.

The first was a libel action against a small Swiss action group, AgDW – Third World Action Group. In 1974 a UK charity, War on Want, had published a report *The Baby Killer* (Muller, 1974). It concentrated largely on the activities of two companies in Africa, the Dutch company Cow & Gate and the Swiss company Nestlé, and it attracted widespread media attention, prompting questions in the British parliament.

Cow & Gate responded to the report quickly. It investigated the matter and formally offered to withdraw its products from sale and distribution, only to be told by government authorities and paediatric experts that such action was not the solution.

The Managing Director of Nestlé, Arthur Furer, also took the report seriously initially and admitted that the whole problem needed to be rethought. But then a German translation of the report was published by AgDW, under the title 'Nestlé kills babies'. The company retaliated fiercely, filing libel charges on four counts: the title; the allegation that its practices were unethical; the allegation that it caused the death of thousands of babies; and the assertion that it employed sales representatives dressed like nurses (the 'milk nurses').

The company offered to settle out of court provided that the group apologized and guaranteed not to spread further accusations. AgDW refused to be silenced and preferred to go to trial. Just before the third and final hearing Nestlé withdrew three of the charges, leaving only the complaint about the title. The judge found the 30 members of AgDW guilty of libel, but fined them a token sum of 300 Swiss francs (US$ 150) each.

Although in terms of criminal law, Nestlé could not be held responsible for intentional killing, its methods and practices were publicly condemned. In his summing up the judge stated (SAFEP, 1976):

> *If the complainant in future wants to be spared the accusation of immoral and unethical conduct, he will have to change advertising practices.*

After the trial Nestlé refused to acknowledge that its practices were either immoral or unethical and in a circular to staff, Mr Furer said he had investigated personally the company's marketing practices (SAFEP, 1976):

> *I was able to see that they were normal and usual advertising methods …. We must affirm that we have full confidence in the ethical basis of our actions.*

The second legal action was initiated by a group of nuns, the Sisters of the Precious Blood of Dayton, Ohio, who were shareholders of the US company Bristol-Myers/Mead Johnson, a company that controlled 35% of the US baby milk market, and which also had thriving infant formula sales in the Caribbean and South-East Asia. The Sisters filed a lawsuit in 1976 against Bristol-Myers, because the company was promoting its products aggressively within health-care systems, in particular employing 'milk nurses' to promote the products to mothers. Bristol-Myers steadfastly refused to acknowledge that a problem existed and asserted that it did not sell formula in areas of chronic poverty. The Sisters proceeded to obtain signed, notarized affidavits from witnesses in eighteen countries testifying to the widespread and indiscriminate promotion of Bristol-Myers products in extremely poor areas. The case was eventually settled out of court in 1978 and Bristol-Myers agreed to send a report to its shareholders which included the evidence collected by the Sisters. The company also agreed to halt all direct consumer advertising and the use of 'milk nurses'.

Both legal cases were significant in raising awareness of the need for greater corporate responsibility. They also strengthened the links between NGOs and health workers in many different countries. But while they gave strong warnings to all the companies that the spotlight could, at any time, be turned on them, the legal actions did not actually fundamentally change the practices of either company. Soon after the announcement that its 'milk nurse' service would be stopped, the General Manager of Bristol-Myers in the Philippines admitted that all but one nurse had been rehired as 'medical representatives' (ICCR, 1982).

It was frustration at the lack of progress in preventing the companies' promotion which led to another development in 1977, a campaign of action that would be described by the companies as "considerably harsher than the most libellous of tracts" (McComas *et al.*, 1983).

In 1977 a small group of people in Minneapolis decided to launch a consumer boycott against Nestlé, with one basic demand: that the company halt all promotion of breast-milk substitutes to parents and health workers, including direct advertising to consumers, the distribution of free samples, and the use of company 'milk nurses'.

Ever since Nestlé had first started to export its 'Milk Food' to the colonized world in 1873, it had cornered and dominated half the global market in baby foods. Nestlé was more able than any other single company to set market trends and influence company behaviour, and its marketing strategies have had a powerful influence on health practices in all parts of the globe. Nestlé's persistent refusal to stop promoting its baby milk has made it the principal target of criticism ever since the trial.

The first boycott (1977–1984) captured the imagination of the public and eventually spread to ten countries. Nestlé was the largest food company in the world, so its heavily promoted products, such as instant coffee and chocolates, were an easy target for consumer action. The success of the boycott was substantial, not only because of its direct economic effects – an estimated US\$ 1070 million in lost sales (Buffle, 1986) – but also because of the damage to the corporate image, the impact on management morale, and the indirect costs of management time and attention spent trying to combat it. When the first boycott ended it was described as "the most important victory in the history of the international consumer movement" (Petersen, 1984).

As a result of the publicity generated by the boycott and the two trials, a US Senate Hearing was held in 1978 in which company representatives faced tough questioning. However, it was clear that little would be achieved without an international solution. Dr Halfdan Mahler, Director-General of WHO, was asked by the US Senate to convene an international meeting. As a result the WHO/UNICEF Meeting on Infant and Young Child Feeding took place in October 1979.

THE DEVELOPMENT OF *THE CODE*
The idea of a code of marketing had been proposed by the International Organization of Consumer Unions (IOCU) in 1971, and was raised at the 1974 World Health Assembly, but it was not until the 1979 meeting that it was really pursued. That it happened then was largely due to the presence of the NGOs at that meeting. In addition to representatives from the UN agencies and governments, 28 people were invited to represent the concerns of charities, church groups, mother support groups, and health professional bodies. These included agencies such as OXFAM, War on Want, the Christian Medical Commission, the Interfaith Centre for Corporate Accountability, La Leche League, The International Confederation of Midwives, and the International Paediatric Association. Also invited were 26 people to represent the industry. During the meeting the decision was reached that a code of marketing should be drawn up and presented to the World Health Assembly.

Protracted negotiations followed, with industry and the NGOs pulling in opposite directions. Regrettably, WHO and UNICEF fell into the role of mediators, rather than leading this vital action for health. Finally, a compromise between all the parties was reached and, at the World Health Assembly of 1981, the *International Code of Marketing of Breast-milk Substitutes* was adopted, with 118 countries voting in favour, 3 abstaining, and only 1 country, the United States, voting against it (WHO, 1981). Although inevitably the product of compromise, this unique document broke important new ground. It was hailed as a major breakthrough and it presented the infant-feeding industry with both a dilemma and a challenge. It was, and is, very different to the codes that companies are used to. Company codes of practice are generally designed to give the appearance of protecting the interests of the consumers, but their primary aim is to protect the interests of the manufacturers (Hamilton and Whinnett, 1987). This *Code*, however, had been initiated and drafted on behalf of the consumer. At long last there was a clear message from authoritative bodies that breast-milk substitutes should not be promoted in any way.

Summary of the Main Points of the *International Code of Marketing of Breast-milk Substitutes*

1. No advertising of breast-milk substitutes.
2. No free samples or supplies.
3. No promotion of products through health care facilities.
4. No contact between company marketing personnel and mothers.
5. No gifts or personal samples to health workers.
6. No words or pictures idealizing artificial feeding, including pictures of infants, on the labels of the products.
7. Information to health workers should be scientific and factual only.
8. All information on artificial feeding, including the labels, should explain the benefits of breastfeeding and the costs and hazards of artificial feeding.
9. Unsuitable products should not be promoted for babies.

THE MANUFACTURE OF CONSENT AND THE AVOIDANCE OF *THE CODE'S* PROVISIONS

The baby milk market is a multi-billion dollar operation; with population growth and the opening of new markets, the potential for continued expansion is immense. It is estimated to be worth $6 billion today; however, it has been calculated that if every baby in the world were to be fed artificially for just 6 months, then that market could expand to $36 billion. Although a large number of food and pharmaceutical companies are involved, in fact about a dozen companies based in Europe, the United States, and Japan control the bulk of the market (Chetley, 1986).

Product differentiation between infant formulas is, for the most part, a myth, so success in increasing sales depends entirely on the marketing skills of the company concerned. Thus, the companies with access to the largest promotional budgets are the most able to capture and keep the largest market share. As a consequence, in many countries three or four transnational companies control 90% or more of the market.

During the final drafting of *The Code* the baby food industry had managed to secure a number of important weaknesses which would be exploited to the full in the coming years (for example, *The Code* had ambiguous wording regarding free supplies of baby milks, it allowed the use of company logos on donated educational material, and it gave no clear guidance on appropriate forms of sponsorship). The industry could not, however, erase the unequivocal statements within the text and in its title. *The Code* was international and, most importantly, *all* countries were required to adopt it "as a *minimum* requirement – *in its entirety*" (emphasis added). Article 11 called on manufacturers to ensure, independently of government action, that their "conduct at every level" conformed to its aims and principles.

The companies began immediately to involve themselves in the drafting procedures with governments in individual countries, urging the adoption of voluntary, self-regulated codes, favourable to industry. They tried to exclude NGOs and minimize their influence. In this way the most important provisions of *The Code* concerning marketing and promotion could be neutralized. The industry's confidence at this time is demonstrated in a statement made by Geoffrey Fookes of Nestlé in 1981, that they were "not really worried that any countries will in fact try to implement *The Code* 'in its entirety' or 'as a minimum requirement'," as stipulated by *The Code* (Chetley, 1986).

Once weak national codes were in place they could be endorsed without fear and the industry's conformity to them could be used as evidence of credibility and responsibility – a vital ingredient in such a delicate and sensitive market.

The Philippines provides a good example of how companies have tried to weaken legislation and shows the urgent need for health workers to have up-to-date information and be ready to take up the arguments. In an effort to halt the promotion of bottle-feeding and the damage that it was causing to Filipino babies, in 1986 the government of the Philippines adopted a strong national law to control baby milk promotion and labelling. In 1989 the government proposed to extend that law by introducing an Act requiring both government and private hospitals to adopt policies which allowed mothers and babies to stay together (rooming-in). The four North American and European companies, Wyeth, Nestlé, Abbott/Ross, and Bristol-Myers, who import 99% of the baby milk into the country, joined forces to complain. In a letter to the Senate the companies claimed that the Act was unnecessarily drastic and that (Leber, 1989):

> *in ward situations, especially in government hospitals, roomed-in new-borns will be at greater risk of getting sick because strict aseptic precautions are not usually implemented.*

Fortunately, the health workers and campaigners in the Philippines had access to the latest data on breastfeeding's protective qualities against infection, through their strong links with NGOs and doctors in Europe. If they had not they might have been swayed by these arguments and the Rooming-in Bill might never have been adopted.

TARGETING OF HEALTH WORKERS, AND HOW HOSPITAL PRACTICES DAMAGE BREASTFEEDING

Health workers are an unpaid, but potentially highly effective sales force for infant formula companies. A single health worker can reach hundreds, possibly thousands, of mothers each year, so any expenditure on convincing them to promote a particular brand is likely to reap high returns.

Following the adoption of *The Code*, and the extensive publicity which had surrounded the issue during the 1970s, the companies became more careful about direct advertising. Their marketing departments were devising new, subtler strategies.

The Interfaith Center on Corporate Responsibility (ICCR) has described the sort of deliberate strategy that the US companies used to influence health practices (ICCR, 1982). Abbott/Ross, at that time the world's second largest infant formula company, employed special promotional experts to penetrate hospitals with a sales force paid on commission. These sales representatives cultivated health workers' dependency through the liberal provision of cash, grants, equipment, and paid travel. Abbott/Ross also provided free architectural services to hospitals, imposing designs that built bottle-feeding into the facility, separating mothers and babies into wards and nurseries. They aimed to 'capture the doctor': "Our goal is to make the physician a low pressure salesman for our products" [Abbott/Ross in-house publication, cited by ICCR (1982)]. The strategy made the hospital the platform for sales promotion:

> When one considers that for every 100 infants discharged from the hospital on a particular formula brand, approximately 93 infants remain on that brand, the importance of hospital selling becomes obvious.
> Abbott/Ross training manual cited in ICCR 1982.

The manual also describes how to divide the hospital into penetrable units and "how to sell when you are not allowed on the floor."

Health workers from all over the world are regularly trained in North American and European maternity hospitals [in 1989, 17,000 overseas health workers were trained in British hospitals alone (Department of Health, 1991)]. With the exception of Scandinavia, these Western facilities are saturated with commercial promotion of baby milk and poor breastfeeding practices.

Surveys carried out in Brazil, Tanzania, and Sri Lanka in 1984 found that the more contact mothers had with health services the more likely they were to bottle-feed, and that traditional knowledge was rapidly lost. Moreover, the mothers who received 'breastfeeding instructions only' actually used commercial products most frequently. This seems curious, until one examines the incorrect and authoritarian instructions. Information for all mothers in one maternity facility stated (Marchione and Helsing, 1984):

> Breast milk is the ideal food for your baby in its first months of life. You ought to persist patiently so that your child may get full advantage from breastfeeding. Clean the nipples of your breasts with special care with boricated (2%) or warm water, before and after feeds. Alternate the breast you offer first, letting the baby suckle on each for a maximum of 15 minutes.
> Times: ... Remember: in the intervals between feeds, offer 20–30 g of boiled water or sweet or camomile tea, sweetened with Nide. Note: If before consulting your paediatrician your milk dries up, offer the child a feeding bottle with 'Nestogeno' milk.

INFORMATION OR ADVERTISING?

With infinite resources at their disposal the baby food companies can offer a range of materials which can seem irresistible to the busy, under-resourced health worker.

The Department of Health of the Philippines, for example, had only 2 million pesos a year to cover all health education in the Philippines in 1986. A single transnational company (Nestlé), selling a range of highly processed foods and drinks, had, in comparison, a budget of 240 million pesos (£8 million)for promotion of its products in that country (IBFAN/BUNSO, 1989).

The aim of *The Code* is to ensure that health workers, mothers, and carers receive full and impartial information about all aspects of infant feeding. Many companies produce free booklets about parenting and infant feeding for prospective and new mothers. All carry the company logo and, if the national code permits, advertising for breast-milk substitutes. The companies argue that such literature helps women to make better 'choices' about infant feeding, deliberately confusing advertising with the provision of impartial information. Brand name adverts provide selective information, and project only the qualities that the advertiser chooses to emphasize. [For an example of 'good practice' in providing information for mothers, see the chart prepared by the RCM (1994), which compares the composition of baby milk brands with the composition of breast milk. It includes the anti-infective, anti-bacterial, anti-parasitic, and anti-viral factors in breast milk. It also points out that all formula have the potential for inadvertent deficiencies, excesses, or contamination.]

An evaluation of free breastfeeding materials in Canada in 1993, for example, showed that the commercial material tended to provide negative images for the mother wishing to breastfeed. It frequently listed cautions, such as watching your diet, avoiding alcohol, smoking and medications, and stressed the risks involved if you did not look after yourself when you breastfed your baby (Valaitis and Shea, 1993).

When the bulk of information on all aspects of infant feeding is financed by the baby food industry, the health care system itself can become a key obstacle to breastfeeding and a number of research studies have examined the way that commercial promotion counteracts messages that health workers try to convey. One randomized trial in the United States showed that removing advertising had more impact on improving breastfeeding rates than intensive efforts to train staff in breastfeeding support. It found that (Frank *et al.*, 1987):

> Compared with commercially prepared discharge materials, non-commercial discharge materials consistent with the WHO Code significantly prolonged by more than 2 weeks the duration of exclusive breastfeeding, delaying the introduction of solid foods, and increased the likelihood that infants would still be breastfeeding, at least partially, at 4 months postpartum.

The non-commercial discharge pack was also associated with lower rates of re-hospitalization of infants.

Another study examined the level of knowledge about breastfeeding in health workers in rural maternity units in Ireland. Although those who responded to a self-reporting questionnaire felt that they had adequate knowledge, their answers did not always bear this out.

Ireland is a major producer and exporter of baby milks, and only 31% of Irish babies are ever breastfed. The researchers found that few of the respondents had access to information from sources other than infant formula companies, whose representatives were frequent visitors to all the maternity units. The majority of midwives' continuing education sessions were funded by infant formula companies too. A recurring comment was "The manufacturers tell us you can't get any closer to mother's milk" (Becker, 1992).

Even simple breastfeeding posters, which conscientious health workers might display in order to encourage good practice, can convey unhelpful messages. Company posters distributed in Botswana in 1989, for example, were supposedly designed to promote breastfeeding, but implied that a breastfed baby could suffocate against the breast if incorrectly positioned, showed an incorrect and ineffective sucking position, and recommended a strict feeding schedule.

It is very much in the companies' interests to provide health services with breastfeeding information which carries their logo. Not only does it enhance their image, but it is also profitable. Companies admit that they make most money out of mothers who had intended to breastfeed. This is because women who give up breastfeeding within a few weeks are likely to use breast-milk substitutes for longer than women who choose to bottle-feed from the start. The mother who intends to breastfeed is typically more concerned about nutrition and is more susceptible to the advertising of products that she believes might be advantageous to her baby – expensive sterilizing equipment, specialized formulas, follow-on formulas, baby drinks, and packaged weaning foods, etc. The mother who chooses to bottle-feed from the start is generally more likely to use cheaper substitutes.

The companies also like to talk about breast milk to health workers because they know that it is acknowledged by scientists to be the 'gold standard'. It is very much in the companies' interests to research into breast milk's composition. By adding various components to their products they can make exaggerated claims about their own milk products being the 'closest to breast milk'. No manufacturer ever gives a proper account of the known hazards of artificial feeding (which is a requirement of The Code's provisions); they prefer to convey the message that bottle-feeding is almost as good as breastfeeding – provided the mother follows the instructions and makes up the feeds correctly. Mishaps are blamed on the mother for not following the instructions properly – or on the health worker for not advising her correctly.

Commercial literature often exaggerates the difficulties mothers may have with breastfeeding, and has been successful in promoting the notion that lactation failure is normal. The term 'insufficient milk syndrome' was coined by the US baby food manufacturer Abbott/Ross in the 1980s and is still used everywhere. Despite the fact that there is no evidence that this syndrome really exists, it was cited as a shocking epidemic in an article in the Wall Street Journal in July 1994 (Helliker, 1994):

> Dying for milk – Some mothers, trying in vain to breastfeed, starve their infants ....
> Though the actual number of cases is impossible to determine, 'insufficient-milk syndrome' may occur as much as 5% of the time, affecting about 2000 mothers a year in the US.

This article was soon followed by coverage on prime-time television. Within a few days the breastfeeding rate in a Chicago hospital had fallen from 85–90% to 40% (Action for Corporate Responsibility, 1995). The next month a similar article appeared in a UK newspaper, The Mail on Sunday, telling of a baby who had been rescued from dehydration when his father "became increasingly concerned for his son's health ... intervened on the tenth day and put Ross on supplementary bottle feeds. Ross is now a healthy little boy" (Wilkerson, 1994). Two months later the Wall

Street Journal carried a promotional article for feeding bottles. In this we learned that the father in the UK story was actually the owner of Cannon Rubber of London, the manufacturer of the feeding bottle in question (*Wall Street Journal*, 1994).

THE THORNY QUESTION OF SPONSORSHIP AND GIFTS

Artificial baby milk does have some uses and is not wholly harmful in the way that tobacco is. This means that the question of whether to accept sponsorship from baby food companies has become, for some health workers, very confused. Many doctors do refuse steadfastly, on ethical grounds, to accept industry support for their work or their research, or to attend conferences sponsored by the baby food industry. However, others, especially those in the richer countries, prefer to see such sponsorship as a benign activity.

The Code does permit companies to fund fellowships, study tours, and research grants, *provided they are disclosed* and *provided that they do not constitute "financial or material inducements to promote products* within the scope of this Code" (WHO, 1981). A health worker who has received a grant from a company may genuinely believe that there is no obligation to that company and that the funding in no way affects future decisions or loyalties.

However, the sources of sponsorship of medical research almost invariably influence the type of research that is undertaken, and they may also affect the outcome of that research. The extent to which health workers and professional bodies are financially dependent on the baby food industry is not easy to establish, but it is clear that sponsorship can act as a powerful constraint on the willingness of individuals and organizations to speak out against unethical practices.

In a paper prepared for the Twelfth Annual Meeting of the World Sugar Research Organization, Professor John Reid, Deputy Principal of the University of Cape Town, explained some of the commercial advantages of funding scientists (Reid, 1983):

> *There is a hidden agenda in the research support business. Those who accept your support are often perceived to be less likely to give you a bad scientific press. They may come up with the results that cause you problems, but they will put them in a context in a way that leaves you happier than had they emanated from someone not receiving your support. My own observation and comment is that this hidden effect is powerful – more powerful certainly than we care to state loudly, either from the point of view of the honour in science or in industry. It takes a lot to bite the hand that feeds you: a muzzle is a good insurance against unwelcome bites.*

No one would argue that the baby food industry does not have a legitimate need to carry out research in order to improve the quality of its own products, but when one considers the slowness with which companies have brought their products into line with international recommendations, it seems likely that the industry's need to silence its critics, while gaining a competitive advantage, are the most important motives for conducting and sponsoring research.

Health workers (and governments) often fail to analyse the financial impact of their company 'gifts', which are rarely as philanthropic as they seem. In one UK hospital the baby food company Farley's spent £2000 sponsoring the launch of 'A New Caring Approach to Midwifery'. This may seem generous, but by providing promotional leaflets for the mothers, glossy notice boards, and badges for the midwives, all carrying the company logo, Farley's gained a permanent place in the hospital along with an implicit endorsement of its products. Four thousand babies are born in the hospital every year, but despite the fact that 75% of mothers say they want to breastfeed at the antenatal classes, only 28% breastfeed exclusively once the baby is born. This is a highly desirable market for any formula producer. Bottle-fed babies need approximately two tins per week for the whole of the first year, so the babies from this hospital could generate over £800,000 per year in baby milk sales. Farley's would have recouped its £2000 donation once seven mothers had chosen its brand over that of another competitor.

CREATING NEW MARKETS

The following extract was taken from a radio interview with a regretful ex-consultant who had worked on an advertising project for Nestlé in the mid-1970s. He explained the marketing strategies they devised (Olle, 1989):

> We were having a discussion among executives from various areas including India, and other executives from Kenya, and a small team from Europe [about] the products that would be most penetrative in these marketing areas and it was duly decided that infant baby formula would be probably the most receptive. Mothers are very emotional ... we wanted to use a nursing mother with the youngest possible baby .... The strategy was formed around the idea that mothers had better things to do with their time than nurse their babies.
> Cosmetic issues were also considered fruitful to exploit: we were appealing to the idea that if you nursed your babies you might suffer from what is referred to as 'bosom sag' and that this would be obviated, of course, if you used these marvellous products.

These messages were extremely powerful and still have a global impact today. Companies have maintained existing markets, and have now established themselves within the health care systems of the former centrally controlled economies of Eastern Europe and Central Asia. New baby food factories are being established in countries such as Poland, Kazakhstan, and China.

With a population of 1 billion and 25 million births every year, the potential profits to be made in China are huge. Traditionally, Chinese women have breastfed their babies for an average of one year. But breastfeeding rates have fallen dramatically during the 1980s. Chinese mothers are now complaining that they do not have enough milk, that breastfeeding will ruin their figures, and that they are reluctant to breastfeed in public. The government has identified the main causes to be (WHO, 1991):

> Increased female participation in the labour force, absence of breastfeeding role models due to changing family patterns, the influence of commercial advertising, hospital practices, and health and psychological factors related to social status.

The *Wall Street Journal* reports that (Gull, 1995):

> Multinationals are jostling to get in on the action .... Toy makers reckon the current market for their products in China is about $940 million ... but sales of

products aimed at China's little emperors are soaring, and many industry executives say China's consumer market could outstrip all other world markets in size within the next two decades. Given such enormous potential, foreign companies figure now is the time to begin building brand awareness and educating Chinese consumers about how to use their products. Heinz, for example, runs regular advice columns in major dailies across China aimed at increasing parents' awareness of the importance of good nutrition. The company also gives away a 'Baby Feeding Guide' to hospitals and at sales counters.

It is hard to establish the extent of the influence of the baby food industry. However, there is evidence of companies paying nurses to make up formula and sales representatives giving free supplies of formula to hospitals – in the full knowledge that this encourages the staff to separate mothers and babies at birth and despite an official government edict which was passed in 1992 to ban this practice (Radford and Arts, 1991).

A 1995 report from an international charity working in the Kunming region tells how one company managed to influence Chinese hospital practices. The report describes how, in 1992, the company started to send large quantities of free formula to the local hospitals, how hospital practices changed, and how breastfeeding rates dropped as a consequence. The report describes the lack of knowledge about breastfeeding management and how one hospital does not allow mothers to breastfeed or even see their infants for a full week! Other hospitals in the city allow the mothers to see their infants, but restrict the feed times.

In recognition of the serious threat to infant health in China, the Chinese Ministry of Health has made a commitment to support UNICEF's Baby Friendly Hospital Initiative (BFHI) and in 1994 over 1000 hospitals received Baby Friendly Awards. *The Code* is to become law in China in 1995 and the BFHI includes the elimination of commercial pressures from the health care setting within its *Ten Steps to Successful Breastfeeding* (see Chapter 1, Appendix II, page 19). Hopefully, the enthusiasm shown in the past few years will be maintained and the problems facing this country adequately addressed before it is too late.

THE ROLE OF IBFAN

In the years following the adoption of *The Code*, little would have been done if it had not been for the efforts of citizens groups who continued to monitor the companies' marketing activities and worked to have *The Code* implemented "in its entirety ... as a minimum requirement."

The groups established systems of staying in touch with each other, and formed a network of kindred organizations called the International Baby Food Action Network (IBFAN). Since 1981 IBFAN has grown from six groups to over 140 in over 70 countries; some of its publications are listed after the references (see page 76). IBFAN's groups vary in the work they do, but every group observes companies' behaviour, and some carry out co-ordinated campaigns, such as boycotts which focus on one or more companies. IBFAN groups also urge and support governments to take effective action and train health workers in *Code* implementation in many countries. The IBFAN Code Documentation Centre in Malaysia holds regular training courses for government representatives on national code drafting.

Since the adoption of *The Code*, a number of governments have made significant efforts to implement it, often in the face of powerful opposition and interference from companies and vested interests. Government action is reviewed at every alternate World Health Assembly, and since 1981 IBFAN has played an active role in ensuring that the issue is properly addressed. Many governments, although keen to be seen in these forums as protecting health, have still failed to analyse the economic impact of artificial feeding and to grasp the potential of breastfeeding for the conservation of national resources. However, at every successive World Health Assembly, stronger and tighter Resolutions are adopted, and at the 1994 Assembly, global consensus on *The Code* was reached for the first time.

THE WAY FORWARD

If the baby food industry is to accept that breast-milk substitutes are special products that must be marketed without promotion, it must receive an unequivocal message from health workers, governments, UN agencies, and consumers that promotion in this area is unethical. Only then will it be concerned enough to stop its harmful practices.

Health workers, especially midwives, play such a key role in the decisions that mothers make that they can never be neutral; they have to decide where they stand. They can either play a role in the protection of infant health or they can assist the growth of the baby milk market. If they want to protect themselves and the mothers and babies in their care the *International Code of Marketing of Breast-milk Substitutes* can be an important tool.

ACKNOWLEDGEMENT

The author would like to express her thanks to Nomajoni Ntombela, Co-ordinator of IBFAN Africa, and to Lisa Woodburn and Gabrielle Palmer for their guidance and support in the writing of this chapter.

REFERENCES

Action for Corporate Accountability (1995) Document the impact. *Action News*, Winter: 10 (citing *ILCA Globe*).

Becker, G.E. (1992) Breastfeeding knowledge of hospital staff in rural maternity units in Ireland. *Journal of Human Lactation*, **8**(3): 137–142.

Buffle, J.C. (1986) *N Comme Nestlé*. Alain Moreau, Paris.

Chetley, A. (1986) *The Politics of Baby Foods. Successful Challenges to an International Marketing Strategy*. Frances Pinter, London.

Department of Health (1991). Personal communication.

Frank, D.A., Wirtz, S.J., Sorenson, J.R., and Heeren, T. (1987) Commercial discharge packs and breastfeeding counselling: Effects on infant-feeding practices in a randomized trial. *Pediatrics*, **80**(6): 845–854.

Gull, S.D. (1995) China's (only) children get the Royal treatment. *Wall Street Journal*, February 2nd.

Hamilton, R. and Whinnett, D. (1987) A comparison of the WHO and the UK Codes of Practice for the Marketing of Breast-milk Substitutes. *Journal of Consumer Policy*, **10**, 167–192.

Helliker, K. (1994) Dying for milk. Some mothers, trying in vain to breast-feed, starve their infants. *Wall Street Journal*, July 22nd.

IBFAN/BUNSO (1989) *Babies Before Profits*. International Baby Food Network and Balikatan at Ugnayang Naglaiayong Sumagip sa Sanggol, The Philippines.

ICCR (1982) Confronting the US infant formula giants. *The Corporate Examiner*. Vol. 11, No. 7–8. Interfaith Center on Corporate Responsibility Infant Formula Program, New York.

Jelliffe, D.B. (1971) Commerciogenic Malnutrition? *Food Technology*, **25**: 55.

Leber, T. (1989) Letter to Marilen Danguilan, Philippines Senate Committee on Health on behalf of Wyeth-Suaco Laboratories, Mead-Johnson Philippines, Nestlé Philippines, Abbott Laboratories (Philippines), and Consolidated Foods Corporation, August 8th.

Marchione, T.J. and Helsing, E. (1984) Results and policy implications of the cross-national investigation: Rethinking infant nutrition policies under changing socio-economic conditions. *Acta Paediatrica Scandinavica*, Supplement 314, 34–43.

McComas, M., Fookes, G., and Taucher, G. (1983) *The Dilemma of Third World Nutrition: Nestlé and the Role of Infant Formula*. Nestlé, Vevey.

Muller, M. (1974) *The Baby Killer: A War on Want Investigation into the Promotion and Sale of Powdered Baby Milks in the Third World*. War on Want, London (2nd edn, 1975; 3rd edn, 1977).

Nestlé (1984) Editorial. *Nestlé News*, February.

Olle, A. (1989) Radio interview, ABC Radio, Australia, October 24th.

PAG (1972) *Promotion of Special Foods (Infant Formula and Processed Protein Foods) for Vulnerable Groups*. PAG Statement No. 23, Protein-Calorie Advisory Group of the United Nations, New York, 18th July (revised 28th November 1973).

Peterson, E. (1984) United Nations Speeches. Peterson was the Consumer Affairs Advisor to United States Presidents Johnson and Carter. United Nations, New York.

Radford, A. and Arts, M. (eds) (1991) *Breaking the Rules 1991*. International Baby Food Action Network/International Organization of Consumers Unions, Penang.

RCM (1994). *Comparison of Breast milk with Infant Formulas Available in the UK*. Royal College of Midwives, London.

Reid, J. (1983) *The Life Cycle of Funding Committees, and the Basis of Committee Decisions*. Paper given at the Twelfth Annual Meeting of the World Sugar Research Organization, Durban, 22-23 March, quoted in O'Connor, M. and Rayner, M. (1993) Sponsorship and health. In: Shaw, R. (ed.) *The Spread of Sponsorship*. Bloodaxe Books, Newcastle Upon Tyne.

SAFEP (1975) *Does Nestlé Kill Babies?* Mimeo, Swiss Information Groups for Development Policy. SAFEP, Berne.

SAFEP (1976) *Nestlé Case Will Not Continue – But Dispute Goes On*. Information for the press, No.5, mimeo, Swiss Action Groups for International Development, unofficial translation. SAFEP, Berne.

Valaitis, R.K. and Shea, E. (1993) An evaluation of breastfeeding promotion literature: Does it really promote breastfeeding? *Revue Canadianne de Sante Publique*, **84**(1): 24–27.

Wall Street Journal (1994) Feeding Baby as Nature Intended. *Wall Street Journal*, October 14th.

Wilkerson, A. (1994) Tiny victims of the 'breast is best' zealots. Scandal of mothers who risk starving their babies. In: Femail on Sunday, *The Mail on Sunday*, August 21st.

Williams, C. (1939) *Milk and Murder*. Address to the Rotary Club of Singapore in 1939. IOCU, Penang, Malaysia.

Williams, C. (1978) Interview. *Lansing Star*, 18th October.

WHO (1981) *International Code of Marketing of Breast-milk Substitutes*. World Health Organization, Geneva.

WHO (1991) *Infant and Young Child Nutrition (Progress and Evaluation Report; and Status of Implementation of the International Code of Marketing of Breast-milk Substitutes).* Report by the Director-General, EB89/28, November 28th. World Health Organization, Geneva.

IBFAN PUBLICATIONS

IBFAN publications include the following:

International Baby Food Action Network/International Organization of Consumers Unions (1981–1994) *Breaking the Rules.* (Regularly produced journals reporting company violations of the *International Code of Marketing of Breast-milk Substitutes.*)

International Baby Food Action Network/International Organization of Consumers Unions (1981–1994) *State of The Code by Country. A Survey of Measures taken by Governments to Implement the Provisions of the International Code of Marketing of Breast-milk Substitutes Adopted by the World Health Assembly in May 1981.* (Charts prepared for the World Health Assemblies.)

International Baby Food Action Network/International Organization of Consumers Unions (1981–1994) *State of The Code by Company. A Survey of Marketing Practices of Infant Food and Feeding Bottle Manufacturers, Compared to the Requirements of the International Code of Marketing of Breast-milk Substitutes.* (Charts prepared for the World Health Assemblies.)

Breastfeeding and Work: The Situation of Midwives and other Women Health Care Providers

Penny Van Esterik

INTRODUCTION

Breastfeeding thrives in family friendly cultures. Unfortunately, few of us work in family friendly institutions. To make the changes necessary for a long-term social transformation, we need a new way of thinking about work and family responsibilities. In many societies, work is seen from a male perspective and valued only if it produces cash income. As much of women's work is home-based or for subsistence, it is under-reported, under-valued, and under-paid. When women also work for a cash income, their work places seldom accommodate their unpaid reproductive work, including pregnancy, breastfeeding, and child care. Most employed women who want to breastfeed give up the ideal of optimal breastfeeding, and resort to partial, mixed, or token breastfeeding after they return to work.

The World Breastfeeding Week in August 1993 offered an opportunity for people world-wide to focus on enabling working women to breastfeed, by taking this as its theme. According to the *Innocenti Declaration* (see Chapter 1, Appendix II, pages 17–18), optimal breastfeeding means that:

> *All women should be enabled to practise exclusive breastfeeding and all infants should be fed exclusively on breast milk from birth to 4–6 months of age. Thereafter, children should continue to be breastfed, while receiving appropriate and adequate complementary foods, for up to 2 years of age or beyond.*

Although every mother is a working woman, it is a particular challenge to assist those who work outside the home to practise optimal breastfeeding. With this in mind, the goals for the campaign were to:

- Enable women to breastfeed with confidence by informing them of the benefits of optimal breastfeeding and of their maternity entitlements.
- Ensure that national legislation to protect the rights of working women to

77

breastfeed is implemented in as many countries as possible.

- Increase public awareness of the benefits of combining work and breastfeeding to women, children, and society at large.
- Encourage trade unions to advocate maternity entitlements that support women workers who breastfeed.
- Foster the establishment of mother-friendly work places everywhere.
- Protect cultural practices which support the breastfeeding mother working at or away from home.

Can we create a woman-centred approach to work that values women's productive and reproductive work, and reduces the double burden that women carry? Such an approach would acknowledge pregnancy, breastfeeding, and child care as socially meaningful and productive work, and recognize the social supports necessary for optimal breastfeeding. Men share the responsibility for providing this support in the home and the work place.

The successful integration of women's productive and reproductive lives is a goal of many women. Our lives reflect the fact that this is not accomplished easily. How many of us recall working on automatic pilot the day after a night with a sick baby, a miscarriage, a teenager's crisis? These normal mothering experiences are unpredictable and uncontrollable, yet they highlight the dilemmas of working mothers who try to keep their reproductive and productive lives neatly separated.

In some parts of the world, the problems of combining breastfeeding and women's work are not solved by individual women, but by communities who offer extra support to women, and assist with child care. Increasingly, however, the Western patterns of social fragmentation and isolation have taken root. The mother finds herself responsible for solving the problem alone, as countries experiencing debt crises and structural adjustment cut back on work-place child care and maternity entitlements. Even in China, where facilities for breastfeeding women at work have for some time included nursing breaks, there are reports of attempts to cut back on these 'frills' in order to increase productivity (Van Esterik, 1992).

The relation between women's productive and reproductive work is more than a scheduling problem – a matter of balancing mother-work with other-work. Women in different societies, different classes, and at different times in their lives accomplish this balancing act in very different ways. But, this is at an increasingly high personal cost as working conditions change. Midwives face these conflicts with particular regularity as their work pattern is determined in part by the reproductive cycles of other women.

During the 1990s, governments have reaffirmed, through the United Nations, the importance and benefits of breastfeeding to infants, mothers, and society at large. In four key documents – the *Innocenti Declaration on the Protection, Promotion, and Support of Breastfeeding* (August, 1990); the *Convention on the Rights of the Child* (September, 1990); the *Declaration of the World Summit on Children* (September, 1990); and the *World Declaration on Nutrition and Plan of Action for Nutrition* (December, 1992) – governments have acknowledged the right of infants and mothers to exclusive breastfeeding; the right of women to correct and consistent information and support in child health and nutrition; and the right of children to protection and development.

These UN documents, together with the International Labour Office (ILO) Conventions on Maternity Protection are minimum standards. They recognize women's rights to maternity and the rights of working mothers to breastfeed their infants. But, in practice, women employed in various work environments face many different obstacles to breastfeeding. For example:

- Maternity leave may only be available to formally employed women on annual or permanent contracts, or only to women working in the public sector.
- In many countries, agricultural workers, domestics, and women working in the informal sector are not covered by existing conventions.
- If costs for leave and child care are borne by the employers alone, they may prefer to hire male workers.
- The lack of adequate income, guaranteed job security, and work-place child care or transportation to community-based care hinder the possibility of breastfeeding, even when maternity leave is available.
- Child care facilities and breastfeeding breaks may be available in large companies, but not in small companies or the informal work settings in which most women work.
- Baby food companies target employed women by promoting their products as the only solution available to working mothers.
- Male-oriented attitudes of governments and employers result in treating maternity benefits as 'doing a favour for women', instead of as an entitlement and an investment in the health of society.
- National socio-economic conditions (e.g., unequal distribution of wealth, poverty, heavy debt financing) leave few resources necessary for health care services to support breastfeeding.
- The overall low social status of women in many countries gives lower priority to women's needs.

WORKING CONDITIONS FOR MIDWIVES

Midwives practise in a wide range of settings – in homes, clinics, hospitals, and other locations. Similarly, the term midwife has been applied to a wide range of practitioners, from traditional birth attendants (TBAs) in developing countries to birth specialists in high-tech hospitals. To a non-professional, all midwives share certain characteristics:

- They are overwhelmingly women (and for the purposes of this chapter I only consider midwives who can breastfeed their own children).
- They are the experts in normal childbirth, who assist women in giving birth in a way that respects their wishes. Thus, mothers are active participants in the birth process with midwives.
- The care they provide continues from pregnancy through birth and postpartum, until (in many societies) the child is weaned from the breast.

This continuity of care for both mothers and infants is one traditional characteristic of midwifery that is rapidly eroding in many urban industrial settings (Rajan, 1993):

Hospital midwives do not see the results of their efforts, as women go home within

*a few days, while community midwives and health visitors are unable to influence
the way in which women first begin to breastfeed ...*

What remains is the ideal that midwives do have a personal, individualized
relationship with their clients. The relationship of respect between midwives and the
mothers they care for stems partly from its historical roots – midwives were most
commonly women elders of menopausal age. Currently, young women of child-
bearing age are entering the profession in large numbers, raising whole new questions
about working conditions within the profession.

The policy statement of the International Confederation of Midwives (ICM)
recognizes a midwife's "unique and vital role in the promotion of breastfeeding at a
governmental, institutional, and individual level" (ICM, 1993). But when midwives
themselves give birth, what support do they have for their own breastfeeding
practices? Here is one experience (Rajan, 1993):

*After delivery I was left to cope alone – presumably I knew all about feeding, being
a midwife myself. Hospital midwives insisted on frequent feeds ... and kept
threatening to give bottled milk if the baby didn't feed.*

Palmer writes (1993):

*It is scandalous that all hospitals do not provide facilities for breastfeeding for
their staff, and, in fact, where this has been done, HPs (health professionals) have
returned earlier from maternity leave thus benefiting the system.*

A midwife who has not been supported in her own breastfeeding may not be the
best support for a new breastfeeding mother. How can she be am effective role model
for other mothers if her own nurturing activities have been curtailed by her working
conditions? One harassed midwife expressed her feelings about being on-call for
other people's babies, often depriving her of time with her own (Campbell, 1990):

*Many's the time I've had to rush off; my own family's gone without. The work
demands a sacrificial sort of love.*

Midwives often seem to communicate mixed messages about breastfeeding,
messages that in some cases reveal their own personal and emotional discomfort with
the intimacy of breastfeeding. One does not have to go far to find manifestations of
this in the midwifery press: comments that "breastfeeding leads to isolation and a very
limited lifestyle" (Scott, 1989), or the following advice (Field, 1984):

*The midwife must not arouse feelings of guilt in the mother who elects to, or must
work, but at the same time she needs to ensure that the mother who decides to stay
home feels as able as her employed counterpart. The midwife must present the
mother with the alternatives she can utilize if she wishes to continue breastfeeding
but still return to work .... Midwives need to discuss with mothers socially
acceptable modes of breastfeeding in public. Although breastfeeding in public is
becoming more commonly acceptable, the woman who sits with her breast openly
exposed in a public restaurant will be intruding on the sensibilities of many people
who certainly do not see this as acceptable dinner-time behaviour.*

The midwives' situation is made even more difficult if they are under pressure from baby food companies, and thus receiving substantial misinformation about infant feeding (Palmer, 1993). Researchers express curiosity as to (Rajan, 1993):

> *Why professional behaviour has remained 'so deeply affected by unfounded assumptions, in spite of the obvious detrimental effect these assumptions have had on breastfeeding'* ...

Yet no mention is made in these studies of the effects of inconsistent and (mis)information about breastfeeding or the powerful vested interests between health professionals and suppliers of commercial baby foods. The 'Ten Point Quality Plan for Midwives in Relation to Breastfeeding' (McDowall, 1991) makes no reference to midwives' relations with sales persons for infant formula. Yet these relations have had a serious effect on hospital practices in many countries. Being a target for industry can be troubling to a young professional, particularly one who has not already experienced childbirth and breastfeeding. When professional training does not emphasize lactation management, then professional, licensed midwives may be at an even greater disadvantage than TBAs in developing countries, or 'granny midwives' in North America.

When health care professionals are convinced of the benefits of breastfeeding and proficient at supporting breastfeeding mothers, one would expect these professionals to develop work place strategies to facilitate the integration of breastfeeding into their own working schedules. This might include support for each other with regard to child care, exchanging shifts, etc. The ICM (1993) states that: "Midwives support and sustain each other in their professional roles, and actively nurture their own and other's sense of self-worth." Has this support extended to breastfeeding support? As Raisler (1993) points out:

> *Providing hospital workers with nursing breaks and a comfortable place to express breast milk helps the breastfeeding health worker to prolong lactation and raises consciousness among hospital staff. After all, if hospitals cannot demonstrate a model of caring for breastfeeding workers, what can be expected from the world of business and industry?*

Some evidence suggests that hospitals are no more accommodating to breastfeeding employees than are other institutions. Other research suggests that hospitals and clinics may have developed useful strategies in this regard. Difficult decisions often have to be made regarding priorities for use of any child care facilities. Some hospitals and other work places give priority to breastfed babies because they are the ones who need frequent access to their mothers. Other work places view this as discriminatory and follow a 'first come, first served' approach.

A hospital in Bangkok has a crèche for infants aged up to a year and a half, so that nursing staff and other employees can breastfeed their babies at their place of work.

A study of the breastfeeding practices of women employees at a hospital in Lagos, Nigeria (Amisaiye and Oyediran, 1983), revealed that women with low salaries breastfed their children for a longer time (8 months) than more senior professional women who breastfed for 3–5 months (mean duration). They recommend a crèche at the place of work and a paid post-delivery leave of 3 months, with the costs shared by the employer and the government.

A hospital in Toronto has a written policy on breastfeeding and offers a private area with an electric breast pump for nursing mothers to use. Mothers buy their own accessory parts for the electric pump, or may provide their own manual pumps, and they are responsible for cleaning them. They can receive advice about breastfeeding from the hospital's Breastfeeding Clinic, which originally existed only for patient use.

In the United States, Katcher and Lanese (1985) found that when facilities were provided for employed breastfeeding mothers in a New Jersey hospital, these mothers were able to combine breastfeeding and hospital employment successfully. The hospital provided 3 months' maternity leave and, on return, time during shifts for expression of breast milk. A refrigerator was supplied for storing breast milk and a breastfeeding consultant was available for advice. In some hospitals, milk banks may be used to assist breastfeeding employed mothers.

Papua New Guinea provides an interesting case study, since the government enacted legislation to make feeding bottles available only by prescription in 1977, and to establish the rights of employed breastfeeding mothers to two half-hour nursing breaks daily during working hours. Marshall's study of the urban public health nursing staff in Port Moresby documents some successful strategies for returning to work and maintaining breastfeeding: the provision of satisfactory child minding near home or near work, allowing public health nurses to transfer to clinics as near to their homes as possible, and allowing young babies to remain in the back room of the clinic (Marshall, 1985).

Lucia Fakudze, a nurse and mother of five children, worked in an occupational health service clinic in Swaziland. After the birth of her fifth child, she was convinced that exclusive breastfeeding was possible for working mothers. With the help of a breastfeeding counsellor, Lucia overcame her problems expressing breast milk and returned to work after 3 months. She was assisted by her helper.

> My helper had never seen the baby get anything else other than breast milk and she was sure that the baby would get sick if he was given any other milk.

The routine of work and breastfeeding was possible because of the policy of the clinic. Lucia says (*SINAN News*, 1989):

> I felt badly at first that I was taking time off to go home and breastfeed mid-morning, but Pat explained that it was the policy of the clinic that the breastfeeding mothers among the staff should be allowed time to go home mid-morning, have an extended lunch hour, and then go home again mid-afternoon.

She easily expressed milk in the evening between feeds, which she stored in the freezer for the times when she was away at work, and her baby grew well and was never sick.

Working in health facilities offers special challenges and special rewards. Most services are financially constrained, and yet the demand to provide consistent excellence in patient care is greater than ever. The need to make the best use of resources is paramount – and the labour resource is central to the achievement of excellence. Women who train as midwives and leave the system to have and care for babies represent a loss to the profession, particularly since midwives who have breastfed successfully themselves are such a special resource to new mothers. Under current conditions, breaks in employment are related to lack of career progress

(Robinson, 1993). How can employers be convinced of the importance of supporting the women who support other women to breastfeed?

THE BOTTOM LINE FOR EMPLOYERS

Employers have to be convinced of the cost–benefit advantage of helping employees to combine breastfeeding and employment. This requires a whole new style of argument for those who are used to discussing the benefits of breastfeeding. Employers are concerned about the direct costs of attracting, hiring, and paying employees, and other real costs, like staff turnover, training, absenteeism, rescheduling, and poor concentration. Personnel managers may be asking how they can attract and retain fully productive workers, and how they can humanize the work place to make it more worker friendly without spending a fortune.

Employers have found that both women and men value a flexible work environment: productivity often rises, as does employee loyalty; staff turnover drops. In addition, studies of midwives' careers in Britain have revealed that midwives want more flexible work hours and crèches (Robinson, 1993). Recognizing this, many hospitals have successfully introduced staggered hours, flexible hours, extended shifts, job-sharing, and other new and creative changes to working conditions. Some even have child care facilities. They may hesitate to commit to further changes, fearing greater costs. But assisting women to breastfeed after they return to work does not entail great costs. Making some of the hospitals' existing patient-centred expertise and resources available to staff, such as access to nutritionists, dieticians, paediatric consultants, and lactation and breastfeeding consultants, and to the related facilities, might be one useful step. Another could be as simple as providing a clean, comfortable and relatively quiet place for mothers to breastfeed or express milk. The institution will not need much space because the number of women employees breastfeeding at any one time is small. All it takes is commitment, positive thinking, and a willingness to be creative and flexible.

A healthy baby is a parent's dream – and it can be an employer's dream too, because parents who lose time from work or who are distracted by parenting concerns are less productive.

Remind the employer of the potential benefits:

- A reduction of the direct and hidden costs of extended leaves, staff turnover, absenteeism, and distraction.
- Fewer last-minute staff changes to accommodate absenteeism or lateness.
- Improvement of the hospital's image in the community as a caring work place where a mother can take breaks to breastfeed her child at a child care centre located at or near the work place, where a care giver can bring a mother's baby in to work for breastfeeding, or where a mother can take breaks to express her milk.
- Reduction in the time of absence from work of the skilled services of a trained and experienced employee.
- Reduced labour replacement and retraining costs.
- Increased employee appreciation and loyalty.
- Flexible schedules allow the institution to extend its hours of operation or service.
- Job sharing can enable employees who cover for each other to acquire new skills.

These are the kinds of arguments that may win you allies in the administration (particularly among administrators who will be themselves enabled to breastfeed or whose wives will be enabled to breastfeed). However, you will need to find supportive allies among other groups as well. Unions have long fought for women's rights in the work place. While an executive might be able to breastfeed in her office, how does this translate down to the lower ranking health workers? Unions have made gains for women, such as longer maternity leaves, but they may need convincing that breastfeeding is an important worker entitlement. Many child care advocates do not want child care at the work place because work sites are not safe enough. Those lobbying for safer work places could well find allies among health workers. ILO Maternity Protection Conventions make provisions for women workers to breastfeed in the work place. Work place safety is an issue that unions, child care advocates, and breastfeeding advocates may be able to collaborate on.

Adequate provision for breastfeeding is an investment in the health of the present and future work-force. Remind your employer that today's babies are tomorrow's workers.

THE BOTTOM LINE FOR BREASTFEEDING HEALTH PROFESSIONALS

Every work context provides different opportunities and constraints for breastfeeding employees. It is impossible to suggest what might be most helpful to midwives in different parts of the world working in different kinds of settings. For this reason, the campaign for mother friendly work places concentrated on essential requirements, rather than the 'ten steps' developed for baby friendly hospitals.

There are three essential requirements to ensure that every mother, regardless of whether she is formally employed or not, can combine breastfeeding and work successfully. These requirements are time, space or proximity, and support. Employers can provide these three requirements for women workers if they have the political will.

Time
- Provide at least 3 months paid maternity leave (with an ideal of 6 months), which begins after the baby is born. Offer other options such as longer maternity leave with partial pay.
- Offer flexible work hours to breastfeeding women, such as part-time schedules, longer lunch breaks, and job sharing.
- Provide breastfeeding breaks of at least 1 hour per day.

Space/proximity
- Support infant and child care at or near the work place, and provide transportation for mothers to join their babies. For rural work sites and seasonal work, use mobile child care units.
- Provide comfortable, private facilities for expressing and storing breast milk.
- Keep the work environment clean and safe from hazardous wastes and chemicals.

Support
- Inform women workers and unions about maternity benefits and provide information to support women's health.
- Ensure that women have full job security.
- Encourage co-workers and management to have a positive attitude towards breastfeeding in public.
- Encourage a network of supportive women in unions or workers' groups who can help women to combine breastfeeding and work.

An example
Of course these guidelines make many assumptions about the kinds of contexts that women work in. But they may be a useful starting point for constructing a list that fits with conditions in your work place. The following set of conditions needed to support breastfeeding women was proposed for an educational institution:

- An affordable infant care centre on or near the work place.
- Centre staff who are supportive and knowledgeable about the needs of breastfeeding working mothers and breastfed infants.
- Daily breastfeeding breaks for workers of up to 1 h per day according to the ILO legislation.
- Standard paid maternity leave with no penalties in terms of promotion or progress through one's training programme (and no pressure not to take the full 17 week leave because it might interfere with the work of the institution).
- Possibilities for flexible working hours or flexible task assignments while an infant is breastfed exclusively.
- A comfortable, private place to express breast milk.
- Access to a refrigerator.
- A network of supportive women in unions or workers' groups who would help women to combine breastfeeding and work.
- An accepting and supportive atmosphere for breastfeeding (and, when occasion demands, babies) in public spaces.
- Access to information and advice on combining breastfeeding and work.

SMALL STEPS
No other institutions are under the obligation to be 'mother friendly' in the same way as hospitals are expected to become 'baby friendly' to conform to the *Ten Steps to Successful Breastfeeding* (UNICEF/WHO, 1989) – see Chapter 1, Appendix II, page 19. It is critically important to insure that hospitals and clinics set community standards for mother-friendly work places, or at least meet the minimal breastfeeding needs of their employees.

For some midwives, these guidelines and suggestions will seem minimal indeed, if they live and work in societies that consider breastfeeding a natural part of life, and accommodate breastfeeding everywhere. These same guidelines and suggestions may seem utopian dreams for other midwives who struggle for job recognition, security, and a living wage. Some of the steps that follow could be taken by individuals, others by local groups, others by national and international associations. Consider what you can do to promote breastfeeding at the work place.

- Raise the issue of breastfeeding at your trade union, women's group, or community organization.
- Self-employed women can form child care co-operatives, even breastfeeding each other's babies.
- Develop co-operative child care programmes at work. Ensure that child care workers are supportive of and knowledgeable about breastfeeding.
- Demand a clean working environment, safe from occupational hazards (e.g., chemicals, radiation), especially for breastfeeding mothers.
- Lobby for adequate paid maternity leave, breastfeeding breaks, and family programmes that include prenatal education about breastfeeding.
- Demonstrate that mother friendly work places are beneficial to all women, and all workers.
- Create alliances with international labour federations to support the rights of breastfeeding workers.
- Inform working women about the advantages of exclusive breastfeeding and the dangers of bottle-feeding.
- Offer practical advice on combining work and breastfeeding to employers and working women.
- Provide family planning methods that support breastfeeding.
- Help employed mothers realize that they can breastfeed without having to resort to commercial products.
- Encourage an accepting and supportive atmosphere for breastfeeding (and, when occasion demands, babies) in public spaces.
- Offer training to child care staff about the needs of breastfeeding working mothers and breastfed infants.
- Research successful strategies that working breastfeeding mothers have used at your work place, and identify features that make work and breastfeeding compatible.
- Locate a comfortable, private place to express breast milk. Add comfortable chairs to women's washrooms (or, better yet, perhaps our most vulnerable members of society should not have to eat in the bathroom).
- Inform occupational health staff about the importance of breastfeeding so that they can be alert for health hazards in work environments, and become advocates for breastfeeding mothers.
- Form a mother support group at your work place to exchange practical information on breastfeeding techniques and management, or join an existing mother support group.
- Publicize the breastfeeding support group and other breastfeeding resources in a newsletter or flyer.
- Consider making a breast pump available for women who leave expressed breast milk at home for their infants.
- Produce an information pamphlet on breastfeeding at work. Include information on the right of employees to take breastfeeding breaks and the right of all women

to breastfeed in public; who to contact if you feel that you are discriminated against because you are pregnant, or breastfeeding, or with a child; the contact person for the breastfeeding support network; the location of a place at work for women who want to breastfeed or express and store milk; availability of day care and infant care near or at the work place.

• Make the pamphlet available to pregnant workers through personnel offices, labour relations offices, health services, and benefits offices.

HIDDEN BENEFITS

Midwives are the first to confirm that breastfeeding meets a baby's nutritional and emotional needs for the first 4–6 months, and continues to contribute to the baby's nutritional health into the second year and beyond; that breastfed babies have stronger immune systems and are healthier than those who receive breast-milk substitutes: and that breastfeeding can save the lives of thousands of children who presently die every year from diarrhoea and acute respiratory infections.

Perhaps it is time to stress what breastfeeding can do for women. When women are supported in their nurturing functions, breastfeeding encourages their confidence and self-reliance, as they are able to provide quality care for their children. Breastfeeding strengthens the bonding relationship between mother and child. This is particularly important for women whose work separates them from their children. Women who have breastfed are less likely to develop breast and ovarian cancers, and have less osteoporosis later in life. These are not the reasons that most women would give for why they breastfeed, but they may be reasons cited by health professionals. After all, it would be difficult to face hospital accountants and cite joy and pleasure as reasons for supporting breastfeeding in the work place.

ACKNOWLEDGEMENTS

This chapter was prepared with the assistance of Maggie MacDonald, a doctoral candidate in the Department of Anthropology, York University. I have made use of documents produced for WABA on the Mother Friendly Work Place Initiative (WABA, 1993), as well as an unpublished brochure prepared for WABA by Cynthia Webster on hospitals as humanized work places.

REFERENCES

Amisaiye, A. and Oyediran, O.(1983) Breastfeeding among female employees at a major health institution in Lagos, Nigeria. *Social Science and Medicine*, **17**(23): 1867–1871.

Campbell, A. (1990) Midwife on trial. *East West Journal*, March: 60–66, 114–115.

Field, P.-A. (1984*) Breastfeeding at Work and Nursing Facilities in Public Places.* Breastfeeding: a challenge for midwives, Seminar and Workshop, Imperial College of Science and Technology, London, UK.

ICM (1993) Position/policy statements adopted by ICM Council at meetings in Vancouver, May 1993. *Midwifery*, **9**: 169–172.

Katcher, A. and Lanese, M. (1985) Breastfeeding by employed mothers: a reasonable accommodation in the work place. *Pediatrics*, **75**(4): 644–647.

Marshall, L. (1985) Wage employment and infant feeding: A Papua New Guinea Case Study. In: Hull, V. and Simpson, M. (eds), *Breastfeeding, Child Health, and Child Spacing: Cross Cultural Perspectives.* Croom Helm, London.

McDowall, J. (1991) The ten point quality plan for midwives in relation to breastfeeding. *Midwives Chronicle and Nursing Notes*, December: 361–363.

Palmer, G. (1993) Who helps health professionals with breastfeeding? *Midwives Chronicle and Nursing Notes*, May: 147–156.

Raisler, J. (1993) Promoting breastfeeding among vulnerable mothers. *Journal of Nurse-Midwifery*, **38**(1): 1–3.

Rajan, L. (1993) The contribution of professional support, information and consistent correct advice to successful breastfeeding. *Midwifery*, **9**: 197–209.

Robinson, S. (1993) Combining work with caring for children, findings from a longitudinal study of midwives' careers. *Midwifery*, **9**: 183–196.

Scott, H.R. (1989) Breastfeeding: Not all romance. *Midwives Chronicle and Nursing Notes*, December: 413–414.

SINAN News (1989) Working at breastfeeding. *Newsletter 3*, Swaziland Infant Nutrition Action Network.

Van Esterik, P. (1992) *Women, Work and breastfeeding*. Cornell International Nutrition Monograph No. 23, Division of Nutritional Sciences, Savage Hall, Cornell University, Ithaca, New York.

WABA (1993) *Mother Friendly Work Place Initiative*. Action Folder for World Breastfeeding Week, 1993, Penang, Malaysia.

CHAPTER 8

Achieving Mother and Baby Friendliness – The Evidence for Labour Companions

G. Justus Hofmeyr and V. Cheryl Nikodem

INTRODUCTION

This chapter considers the way in which the medical model of care in childbirth has eroded traditional mechanisms of support for women. The authors review the evidence from randomized trials on labour companionship that have been conducted in different countries in recent years. They conclude that there is incontrovertible evidence concerning the importance of providing a supportive environment to enable women to achieve their potential, both in terms of the physical process of childbirth and the emotional adaptation to the demands of parenthood.

MEDICAL CONTROL OF CHILDBIRTH AND THE LOSS OF SELF-DETERMINATION

During the twentieth century, remarkable changes have occurred in the circumstances surrounding childbirth for communities with access to western medical facilities. In the first instance, these changes have involved increasing medical involvement in the process of childbirth, which has changed from a primarily home-based active experience with intensive support for the child-bearing woman from members of her community, to a largely hospital-based process controlled by medical personnel. In 1920 in the first issue of the *American Journal of Obstetrics and Gynecology*, DeLee wrote that the objective of obstetric care should be for all nulliparous and most multiparous women to labour under 'twilight' analgesia and be delivered by a specialist obstetrician under general anaesthesia with the routine use of forceps and episiotomy (DeLee, 1920).

The increasing medical involvement in the process of childbirth has been associated with important improvements in maternal and perinatal mortality and morbidity rates. Similar improvements occurred in countries, such as the Netherlands, in which medical intervention was limited to women with specific complications of pregnancy. These observations suggest that for many women, certain medical interventions which have tended to become routine may be unnecessary. Randomized trials of the routine use of many of the individual elements of medical intervention in childbirth have failed to demonstrate their effectiveness or, indeed, have found them to be harmful (Chalmers, 1989).

Reaction to excessive medical intervention in childbirth occurred to varying extents in different communities during the second half of the twentieth century. Such reaction has often been consumer-driven by women organizing themselves to demand change, or led by individual 'maverick' medical professionals.

Of particular concern is the loss of self-determination which women may experience in a hospital environment. Responsibility for care is assumed by medical and nursing staff, on whom the women are dependent for their most basic needs. The relegation of mothers in hospitals to the role of patients receiving care may undermine their sense of personal achievement, and this loss of personal control is accentuated during labour when women are most vulnerable.

THE IMPORTANCE OF SOCIAL SUPPORT DURING LABOUR

One of the most profound ways in which the hospital-based, medical approach has changed the process of childbirth has been the isolation of labouring women from supportive female companionship, which has been a feature of virtually every pre-industrialized society that has been studied (Kennel and Klaus, 1988). Little attention appeared to be given to the possible effects of these changes on labouring women. Reports of studies designed to investigate such possibilities did not, to our knowledge, appear before the 1980s. However, serendipitous evidence emerged from other studies suggesting that emotional support during labour may be of importance. Two examples of such suggestive evidence follow.

In *Practical Obstetric Problems*, Ian Donald (1969) wrote of the use of the abdominal decompression suit during labour:

> *The claims of the Johannesburg workers have been investigated by Loudon in Edinburgh. He came to the conclusion that the beneficial effects were to some extent attributable … to the interest of those handling the apparatus and conducting the experiment, which may, indeed, be a sad reflection on the hunger for care which women in labour experience in our labour wards.*

During the 1970s, the care of women during labour was greatly influenced by the impressive results reported by O'Driscoll employing 'active management of labour' (O'Driscoll *et al.*, 1969; O'Driscoll and Maegher, 1980). Obstetricians paid considerably more attention to the medical aspects of this policy, such as early use of oxytocin, than to the emphasis placed by O'Driscoll on the fact that women were guaranteed the continuous presence of a consistent companion, usually a pupil midwife, throughout their labour. Several authors have suggested recently that this intensive support may have had as much to do with the impressive results reported as the ready use of oxytocin.

By the 1980s, direct evidence of the importance of labour companionship began to appear. In two studies conducted in Guatemala, women from a rural background giving birth in a busy, Western-style hospital, were randomly assigned to receive continuous companionship from a lay worker, or *Doula*, or to act as controls (Sosa *et al.*, 1980; Klaus *et al.*, 1986). Those who received support from a *Doula* experienced considerably shorter labours and fewer caesarean sections. To explain such striking results, it has been suggested that the stress of labour in an unsupportive environment may result in excessive catecholamine secretion. In animal studies, environmental disturbance has been shown to have a negative effect on uterine contractions and placental blood flow, probably as a result of catecholamine release. There is some evidence that similar mechanisms may operate in humans (Lederman *et al.*, 1978).

The Guatemalan studies raised several important questions. Were the results a function of the extreme degree of dislocation and isolation normally experienced by the population studied, who were described as women from a rural background subjected to an unfamiliar Western-style hospital environment, or would they be applicable to women giving birth in a familiar community hospital? Would the effects of companionship be measurable in terms of circulating levels of stress hormones? Might there be longer-term benefits with respect to the women's adaptation to parenthood and relationship with their families?

THE CORONATION HOSPITAL STUDY

To investigate these questions we undertook a prospective randomized control trial of labour companionship at Coronation Hospital in the western suburbs of Johannesburg. Our hypotheses were, first, that labour in a hospital environment may affect adversely the progress of labour and be associated with increased stress-hormone secretion; and second, that the process of relegating women to the position of patients may deprive them of the sense of self-esteem and self-confidence which might otherwise result from taking responsibility for and coping with the birth process, and that this loss of self-esteem might impair their capacity for confident parenting and breastfeeding. We proposed that the above adverse effects of the clinical labour environment may, to some extent, be reversed by the provision of supportive labour companionship.

Coronation Hospital is a University/State hospital serving an economically and, at the time of the study, politically disadvantaged community in the western suburbs of Johannesburg. Many of the women who gave birth in the hospital were young unmarried mothers. It was unusual for women in labour to be accompanied by a support person.

It may be argued that labour companionship should be provided by someone known to the woman, or whom she has met in the antenatal period, who will be with her throughout labour, and continue to provide support during the neonatal period. However, in order to achieve effective randomization and minimize the chance of withdrawals, we limited the intervention in our study to a defined period of companionship commencing, after randomization, in established labour until the birth of the baby. We were aware that this limitation was likely to underestimate the potential effects of companionship, but chose this route to ensure that if benefits were detected, they could reliably be ascribed to the intervention, owing to the tightness of the study design. The objective was thus to determine in principle whether labour companionship conferred certain benefits, rather than to measure the full extent of such benefits given optimal companionship.

It was decided that the companions should not have any medical or nursing background. The first reason for this was that the objective was to assess the effects specifically of companionship. If the companions were trained nurses, it would not be clear whether any effects measured were due to companionship or to professional help with aspects of the labour. Also, it was felt that a companion with nurse training might tend to carry out nursing functions rather than concentrating entirely on the objective of providing emotional support. Third, it was thought that women who were uncomfortable with the hospital environment might identify a nurse supporter with the medical establishment, whereas a lay supporter from a similar background might be perceived as someone less intimidating and easier to relate to.

Advertisements were placed in local churches asking for applicants to act as labour companions. It was explained that the work would be voluntary, but that a small allowance would be paid to cover expenses. Twenty women responded. They were interviewed first in a group and the study was explained to them all. Thereafter, they were interviewed individually. Using discussion and role play of a labour scenario, their intrinsic warmth of personality and ability to convey feelings of empathy were evaluated. Two supporters were selected, and two others asked to act as reserves, one of whom subsequently also took part in the study. All three companions who participated in the study were older women with grown-up children of their own. They expressed a strong desire to help young women during childbirth. They received no formal training other than careful explanation of what was expected of them. They were asked to use their personal resources to help and support the women to whom they were allocated by being present, talking to them, and holding them. They were asked to concentrate on three aspects of support: comfort, reassurance, and praise. The last was emphasized because of our hypothesis that one of the ways in which the medical environment may interfere with a mother's development of the self-confidence needed for parenting is by providing care which minimizes the role of the mother in the birth of her child.

The study design was a randomized control trial. The objective of such a trial is to study two groups of women who are similar in every way except with respect to the intervention being studied. As it is not possible to measure every characteristic which might influence the outcomes being measured, the balance between the groups is achieved by allocating women absolutely at random to the support group or the control group. To avoid any chance of bias in the results, when a woman is selected and entered into the study, the researcher must have no idea to which group she will be allocated. Once entered into the study, the woman is allocated to a group by a random method. At the end of the study, the results of each woman must be counted together with the group to which she was originally allocated, whether or not it has been possible to conform to the management for which she was allocated. Those measuring the outcomes should as far as possible not know to which group each woman belongs.

The study was performed as follows. Women who were having their first child and were in established labour with no complications and without a companion were asked to participate in the study, which was carefully explained to them. If they agreed, they signed consent to participate. A short baseline questionnaire was administered and baseline physiological measurements were made and blood specimens collected. Thereafter, they were allocated to one or other group by opening the next in a series of sealed envelopes containing allocation cards in random order (no pattern to the order). Those allocated to the control group continued with routine care. Those allocated to the support group, in addition to the routine care, were accompanied for the rest of the labour by one of the labour companions.

The physiological measurements were repeated 1 h after entry into the trial and blood was again collected to measure stress hormones. After the birth, blood was collected from the mother and from the umbilical cord and details of the labour were recorded. The day after the birth a questionnaire was administered to assess the woman's response to the labour, her attitude to her baby, and her feelings of anxiety and self-esteem. At 6 weeks and, again, 1 year after the birth a similar questionnaire was completed, including assessment of feeding practices, her relationship with her partner, and any feelings of depression.

The results of the labour outcome and the assessments at 6 weeks and 1 year are presented, together with the results from other randomized trials of labour support.

RESULTS OF THE CORONATION HOSPITAL LABOUR SUPPORT STUDY

Our hypothesis consisted of two distinct stages. First, that the hospital environment may have a negative effect on the progress of labour and on the psychological process whereby a woman gains the self-esteem to respond positively to the labour and to have confidence in herself as a mother and her ability to breastfeed. Second, that this negative effect may, to some extent, be overcome by the provision of supportive companionship with an emphasis on comfort, reassurance, and praise for the labouring woman.

At the time of enrolment into the study in early labour, the study group that received continuous companionship (92 women) had very similar characteristics to the control group (97 women), as the allocation to each group was entirely at random. Therefore, any difference in outcome between the two groups could be ascribed with some confidence to the support provided for the women in the study group.

The major findings of the Guatemala studies (Sosa *et al.*, 1980; Klaus *et al.*, 1986) were a large reduction in the duration of labour and the rate of caesarean section in the supported group (*Figure 8.1*). In the Coronation Hospital study, differences in

Reference	Epidural use (%)		Labour length (h)		Caesarian (%)	
	Support/Control		Support/Control		Support/Control	
Sosa *et al.*, 1980, Guatemala	–	–	8.8	19.3 $p < 0.001$	19%	27%
Klaus *et al.*, 1986, Guatemala	–	–	7.7	15.5 $p < 0.001$	7%	17% $p < 0.01$
Hodnett and Osborn, 1989a, Toronto	61%	80% $p < 0.02$	8.9	8.5 NS	17%	18% NS
Kennell *et al.*, 1991, Houston	7.8%	55.3% $p < 0.0001$	7.4	9.4 $p < 0.0001$	8%	18% $p < 0.01$
Hofmeyr *et al.*, 1991, Johannesburg	–	–	9.6	10.2 NS	12%	14.4% NS

Figure 8.1 Labour outcome in randomized trials of labour companionship.

these physical outcomes of labour were small and not statistically significant. The studies from Guatemala suggested that the crowded, impersonal hospital environment may have been so unfamiliar and threatening to the women in the study that anxiety-related stress-hormone secretion may have interfered with progress in labour in the control group and been ameliorated in those who received support. It may be that the environment in our study, a community hospital familiar to the women in the study, may have been less threatening than that of the Guatemala studies, and therefore provided less scope for improved physiological outcome related to support. The relatively late entry point in the Coronation Hospital study (well-established labour) may also have limited the scope for effect on the duration of labour, particularly the latent phase of labour.

Another study of labour support in which the duration of labour and caesarean section rates were reduced significantly in the support group was carried out in Houston in the United States (Kennell *et al.*, 1991). In that study, epidural analgesia was used significantly more frequently in the control group (*Figure 8.1*). The use of epidural analgesia may possibly have contributed to the longer labours in the control group (the second stage of labour, in particular, may be increased with epidural analgesia).

In contrast to the limited effect of labour support on the physiological progress of labour in the Coronation Hospital study, the psycho-social effects were striking. Comparison of the results of structured questionnaires administered 24 h after delivery showed that, compared with the control group, the support group reported a more positive experience of labour, they had undertaken more activities with their babies, and their state (current) anxiety scores (Spielberger, 1983) were lower (Hofmeyr *et al.*, 1991; Wolman, 1991).

Three-quarters of the participants in the study were interviewed again 6 weeks after the birth. Those who had received continuous support during labour displayed significantly lower state anxiety scores, higher self-esteem scores (Coopersmith, *et al.*, 1967), more facilitative parenting practices (Raphael-Leff, 1985), lower depression scores (Pitt, 1968), more positive relationships with their partners, and longer exclusive breastfeeding periods (Hofmeyr *et al.*, 1991; Wolman, 1991; Wolman *et al.*, 1993).

In order to assess longer-term outcomes, additional subjects were enrolled into the study. One year after the birth it was possible to interview about half of the original groups. Although the result trends were similar to those found at 6 weeks, in most cases the differences were no longer statistically significant. An exception to this was the relationship between the women and their partners. Fewer women in the supported group felt that their relationship with their partner had deteriorated since the birth of the child. Significantly fewer in the supported group had failed to resume sexual intercourse within 3 months of the birth (Nikodem, 1993).

The importance of the above results is that they establish the principle that the human environment during childbirth can have a profound effect on a woman's self-confidence and ability to adapt positively to the demands of becoming a mother. We need to recognize childbirth as a time of unique psychological sensitivity. Women who feel that they have coped well with the demands of childbirth may carry the sense of self-confidence into the early days and weeks of parenting, with a self-perpetuating positive effect on their family interaction and ability to breastfeed successfully. We need to conceptualize childbirth not as a physiological event culminating in the birth of a child, but as a vital and vulnerable period in the continuous process of becoming a mother.

WORLDWIDE TRIALS OF THE EFFECTS OF CONTINUOUS SUPPORT FROM A LABOUR COMPANION

Hodnett (1994) reviewed the results of 11 trials in which women were allocated randomly to have the continuous presence of a labour companion, or to receive routine care only (the control groups). The trials took place in Guatemala, Finland, South Africa, Canada, France, Belgium, Greece, and the United States. The women studied varied from relatively poor women giving birth in a crowded hospital environment in Guatemala to more affluent women in hospitals with access to interventions such as epidural analgesia. In some of the studies the women were also accompanied by their husband, partner, or a family member; in these studies the companionship was provided by a specific professional nurse or midwife who was present continuously, as opposed to the intermittent care received by women in the control groups. In the remaining studies the women were not accompanied by a family member, usually because this was not the norm in the particular hospital, and in most of these the continuous companionship was provided by a lay worker, such as those described in the Coronation Hospital study. Despite these differences, the trials were analysed together because of the general consistency of their results.

Selected results from the 11 trials are shown in *Figure 8.2*. The odds ratio indicates the occurrence of a particular problem in the supported groups compared to the control groups. The 95% confidence interval indicates the range within which the true odds ratio can, with 95% certainty, be expected to lie. If the whole 95% confidence interval falls below 1, there is at least a 95% level of certainty that a true difference exists between the two groups. In other words, a statistically significant

Outcome	No. of trials	Support group	Control group	Odds ratio	95% confidence interval
Epidural analgesia used	4[a]	390/1073	479/1068	0.70	0.59–0.83
Any analgesia	9[a]	525/1493	645/1576	0.68	0.58–0.79
Problems during labour	1[a]	45/186	141/279	0.33	0.23–0.49
Forceps or vacuum deliveries	10[a]	289/1801	368/1939	0.73	0.62–0.88
Perineal trauma	1[a]	56/72	67/73	0.34	0.14–0.84
Caesarian delivery	10[a]	107/1526	174/1679	0.72	0.56–0.92
5 minute Apgar scores <7	7[a]	17/1457	33/1434	0.50	0.28–0.87
Severe labour pain reported	3[a]	128/881	141/892	0.87	0.63–1.21
Labour experience not very satisfactory	3[a]	101/1001	136/995	0.67	0.50–0.89
Finding mothering difficult	1[a]	59/92	89/97	0.20	0.10–0.40
Non-exclusive breastfeeding at 6 weeks	1[b]	36/74	53/75	0.39	0.19–0.81
High depression score at 6 weeks	1[c]	0/74	16/75	0.00	0.00–0.22
Resume intercourse after 3 months	1[d]	44/63	57/65	0.33	0.12–0.88

[a]Hodnett, 1994; [b]Hofmeyr et al., 1991; [c]Wolman et al., 1993; [d]Nikodem, 1993.

Figure 8.2 Selected results from 11 trials in which women were allocated randomly to either receive continuous companionship during labour or routine care only (control group).

improvement was seen in the supported groups with respect to epidural analgesia use, any analgesia use, 'problems' during labour, forceps or vacuum deliveries, perineal trauma, caesarean delivery, 5 minute Agpar scores, satisfaction with the labour experience, satisfaction with the mothering experience, breastfeeding at 6 weeks, depression at 6 weeks, and resumption of intercourse.

It is clear from *Figure 8.2* that not all the outcomes were measured in all the studies. However, meta-analyses of the results from those studies in which particular outcomes were measured show positive effects on a wide range of the physiological and psychological outcomes listed above. Although many other outcomes not shown in *Figure 8.2* showed less convincing differences, to date no adverse effects of being supported have been found in any of the trials.

IMPLICATIONS OF THE STUDIES OF CONTINUOUS COMPANIONSHIP DURING LABOUR

The studies of the effects of continuous companionship during labour have shown beneficial effects over a wide range of physiological and psychological outcomes. There can be no doubt that companionship during labour is an important and fundamental human need. When it is lacking, labour outcomes are adversely effected. The nature of these effects may vary according to the extent to which the birth environment is experienced as threatening, frightening, intimidating, or unsupported.

Enormous attention has been paid to efforts to ensure the physical safety of mothers and their babies during childbirth. Similar attention needs to be paid to the human environment, which may impact at both a physiological and a psychological level on the outcome of childbirth.

The randomized trials referred to above have used as the supportive companion an unfamiliar person, primarily because such an intervention is amenable to the system of random allocation essential to establish the principles outlined above. Now that the concept of labour companionship has been validated in this way, it should be applied as broadly and creatively as possible, and in ways appropriate to the special needs and restrictions of different childbirth situations. Some of these are dealt with in the following sections.

THE ROLE OF MEDICAL AND NURSING PERSONNEL

The medical approach to childbirth may undermine the woman's sense of competence and achievement. Interactions between medical or nursing staff and women in labour often take the form of controlling activities, such as withholding permission, giving instructions to conform to hospital policy, or being condescending, "Don't worry about anything, we will take care of you." These interactions are in sharp contrast to those of the lay companions in our study. We gave them very little formal instruction, except to ask them to use their intuitive personal resources to express empathy, using words and touch, and to concentrate always on three aspects: comfort, reassurance, and praise.

Our study results suggest that health service personnel should pay particular attention to the needs of labouring women for comfort, reassurance, and praise, and that strategies to achieve this should be incorporated into the training programmes of medical and nursing students.

Some nurses and midwives argue that we should not be bringing lay workers into the labour ward to perform tasks that should be part of the nurse's or midwife's role. We certainly agree that every effort should be made by the nursing staff to provide emotional support. However, in reality nursing and midwifery staff with the best will in the world are often too busy with other nursing functions, and with more than one woman to attend to, to be able to provide the kind of uninterrupted companionship that appears to be of importance. In a work-sampling study of obstetric nursing activities in a Toronto teaching hospital, only 9.9% of the nurses' time was actually spent in supportive care activities and only 0.3% in physical contact in the form of reassuring touch (McNiven et al., 1992).

It is also possible that women in labour, particularly those from disadvantaged communities, may feel in awe of the professional staff and find it difficult to relate to them. Some nursing and midwifery staff may be young and have insufficient life experience on which to draw to provide support during the long hours of labour. In contrast, the lay workers employed in the Coronation Hospital study were older women with personal experience of childbirth. They were selected specifically for their warm personal attributes. They were drawn from the community served by the hospital, and were able to establish a close rapport with the women in their care.

For these reasons, without minimizing the importance of the supportive role of midwives or nurses, we suggest that there are many situations in which lay workers may play a valuable role.

We were also interested to see that the nursing staff at Coronation Hospital, who initially had serious reservations about the introduction of lay companions to the labour ward, quickly became convinced of their value when they saw how effective they were at overcoming the anxiety of the women to whom they were allocated as companions.

SUPPORT FROM HUSBANDS/PARTNERS AND OTHER FRIENDS OR RELATIVES

The move towards family-centred maternity care has placed much emphasis on the supportive role of the women's husbands or partners, and their presence has become the norm in countries such as the UK. Research has shown that women in general rate the support of their husbands highly. However, in one study an objective analysis of the quality and quantity of supportive activities carried out showed that the actual support provided by husbands compared unfavourably with that provided by female supportive companions (Bertsch et al., 1990). Men obviously vary in their capacity to provide consistent support. Some may find it difficult to witness the pain experienced by their partner. The presence of a husband or family member may create inhibitions and pressures on the women to meet with behavioural expectations. Pre-existing interpersonal problems may be brought into the labour ward situation. In many cultures, the concept of men being present during childbirth is entirely foreign and unacceptable. For these reasons, the relative anonymity of a female lay supporter may be more acceptable and less threatening to some women than a family member or associate.

Women should be able to have with them during labour whoever they believe will be helpful. Participation in labour preparation classes may help a woman's partner or associate to provide more effective support during labour. We would recommend that in such preparation emphasis should be placed on the triad of comfort, reassurance, and praise. However, it should not be presumed that the partner or associate will always be able to provide sufficient support. Indeed, in one of the randomized trials summarized above (Hodnett and Osborn, 1989b) significant improvements in labour outcome occurred when support from a trained support person was provided over and above the presence of the partner, indicating that on average the support from partners is less than optimal.

CONCLUSIONS: THE WAY FORWARD

As medical and midwifery personnel entrusted with the care of women during childbirth, we have a responsibility to respond appropriately to the evidence from randomized trials concerning companionship during childbirth. First, we need to acknowledge that there is incontrovertible evidence of the importance of a supportive environment to enable women to achieve their potential, both in terms of the physical process of childbirth and the emotional adaptation to the demands of parenthood.

Second, we need to ensure that we place appropriate emphasis on the supportive aspects of our work, both in our day-to-day care of women during childbirth and in the training of students. We need to be particularly sensitive to the potential for routine procedures and attitudes of staff to deprive women in our care of the independence and self-esteem that is of such importance to their ability to give birth and embark on parenthood with confidence.

Third, we need to encourage women who give birth in our hospitals and clinics to be accompanied by those whom they feel are able to comfort and support them during childbirth; and we need to provide training to enable the chosen supporters to be effective in their supportive roles.

And, finally, we need to give serious consideration, in consultation with the communities we serve, to establishing programmes to bring women from the community on a voluntary or paid basis into our hospitals to provide supportive companionship for those women who wish to avail themselves of such support. In doing so, we will need to address the misgivings commonly expressed about members of the public entering labour wards. It should be remembered that similar reservations were expressed previously about partners entering the labour ward, and these problems seem to have been overcome in many countries.

Our experience of advertising for women prepared to act as voluntary labour companions has been an overwhelming response from women who expressed a strong wish to help other women during labour. Many gave as their reason the fact that when they themselves had given birth they had felt the need for support from other women. It seems likely that in most communities there would be women prepared to act as labour companions. It might also be possible in certain communities to draw on the resources of women who have experience of care during childbirth, such as traditional birth attendants. We suggest that in the training of labour companions, a useful starting point may be the functions chosen in the Coronation Hospital study: comfort, reassurance, and praise.

ACKNOWLEDGEMENTS

We acknowledge the contributions to the Coronation Hospital labour support study of Wendy-Lynne Wolman, Beverly Chalmers, Tami Kramer, Daphne Holmes, Katie Koeberg, Norma Schultz, Rose Campbell, Ursula Benjamin, Monica Adams, Lynn Enraght-Moony, Metin Gülmezoglu, the Coronation Hospital Nursing Staff, and the South African Medical Research Council.

REFERENCES

Bertsch, T.D., Nagashima-Whalen, I.Z., Dykeman, S., Kennell, J.H., and Mcgrath, T.S. (1990) Labor support by first-time fathers: direct observations with a comparison to experienced *doulas. Journal of Psychosomatic Obstetrics and Gynaecology,* **11**: 251–260.

Chalmers, I. (1989) Evaluating the effects of care during pregnancy and childbirth. In: Chalmers, I., Enkin, M., and Keirse, M.J.N.C. (eds), *Effective Care in Pregnancy and Childbirth.* Oxford University Press, Oxford.

Coopersmith, S. (1967) *The Antecedents of Self-esteem.* Freeman, San Francisco.

DeLee, L.B. (1920) The prophylactic forceps operation. *American Journal of Obstetrics and Gynecology,* **1**: 34–44.

Donald, I. (1969) *Practical Obstetric Problems.* Lloyd-Luke, London.

Hodnett, E.D. (1994) Support from care givers during childbirth. In: Enkin, M.W., Keirse, M.J.N.C., Renfrew, M., and Neilson, J.P. (eds), *Pregnancy and Childbirth Module. 'Cochrane Database of Systematic Reviews': Review No. 03871,* May: Disk issue 1, 'Cochrane Updates on Disk'. Update Software, Oxford.

Hodnett, E.D. and Osborn, R.W. (1989a) Effects of continuous professional intrapartum support on childbirth outcomes. *Research in Nursing and Health,* **12**: 289–297.

Hodnett, E.D. and Osborn, R.W. (1989b) A randomized trial of the effects of monitrice support during labor: Mothers' views two to four weeks postpartum. *Birth,* **16**(4): 177–183.

Hofmeyr, G.J., Nikodem, V.C., Wolman, W.-L., Chalmers, B.E., and Kramer, T.R. (1991) Companionship to modify the clinical birth environment: effect on progress and perceptions of labour, and breastfeeding. *British Journal of Obstetrics and Gynaecology,* **98**: 756–764.

Kennell, J.H. and Klaus, M.H. (1988) The perinatal paradigm: is it time for a change? *Clinical Perinatology,* **15**: 801–813.

Kennell, J., Klaus, M., McGrath, S., Robertson, S., and Hinkley, C. (1991) Continuous emotional support during labor in a US hospital. A randomized controlled trial. *Journal of the American Medical Association,* **265**(17): 2197–2201.

Klaus, M.H., Kennell, J.H., Robertson, S., and Sosa, R. (1986) Effects of social support during parturition on maternal and infant morbidity. *British Medical Journal,* **29**(3): 585–587.

Lederman, R.P., Lederman, E., Word, B.A., and McCann, D.S. (1978) The relationship of maternal anxiety, plasma catecholamine, and plasma cortisol to progress in labour. *American Journal of Obstetrics and Gynecology,* **132**: 495–500.

McNiven, P. and Hodnett, E. (1992) Supporting women in labor: a work sampling study of the activities of labor and delivery nurses. *Birth,* **19**(1): 3–8.

Nikodem, V.C. (1993) *Companionship to Modify the Clinical Birth Environment: Long-Term Effects on Mother and Child.* RAU (MCur dissertation), Johannesburg.

O'Driscoll, K. and Maegher, D. (1980) *Active Management of Labour.* W.B. Saunders, London.

O'Driscoll, K., Jackson, R.J.H., and Gallagar, J.T. (1969) Prevention of prolonged labour. *British Medical Journal,* **2**: 447–480.

Pitt, B. (1968) 'Atypical' depression following childbirth. *British Journal of Psychiatry*, **114**: 1325–1335.

Raphael-Leff, J. (1985) Facilitators and regulators: vulnerability to postnatal disturbances. *Journal of Psychosomatic Obstetrics and Gynecology*, **4**(3): 151–168.

Sosa, R., Kennell, J.H., Klaus, M., Robertson, S., and Urrutia, J. (1980) The effect of a supportive companion on perinatal problems, length of labor and mother–infant interaction. *New England Journal of Medicine*, **303**(11): 597–600.

Spielberger, C.D. (1983) *Manual for the State–Trait Anxiety Inventory*. Consulting Psychologists Press, Palo Alto.

Wolman, W.-L. (1991) *Social Support during Childbirth: Psychological and Physiological Outcomes*. University of the Witwatersrand (PhD thesis), Johannesburg.

Wolman, W.-L., Chalmers, B., Hofmeyr, G.J., and Nikodem, V.C. (1993) Postpartum depression and companionship in the clinical birth environment: A randomized, controlled study. *American Journal of Obstetrics and Gynecology*, **168**(5): 1388–1393.

CHAPTER 9

In Whose Interest? Women's Experiences of Hospital Birth in Nepal

Maureen Minden

In many countries poor women have no voice. Their social status and their gender combine to make it difficult for them to be heard, yet how else can we know what they need from their maternity services, in the reality of their lives? The study described in this chapter was undertaken because of concern about whether current maternity services were meeting the needs of poor Nepalese women. It was carried out in a large maternity hospital in Kathmandu, and focuses on women's accounts of their own experiences of pregnancy and childbirth, and their perceptions of the services available.

BACKGROUND

Nepal is a small country on the southern slopes of the Himalayas. The population is about 19 million, the annual population growth rate is 2.6%, and the average annual urban growth rate 7.4% (HMG/UNICEF, 1992). Depleting land resources, an increasing population, and the construction of highways have caused a trend in migration to urban areas. The Central Development Region contains about a third of the total population, and here in the mid-mountain area lies the capital city, Kathmandu.

Nepal is one of the world's poorest countries, with an estimated 41.2% of the population living below subsistence level, and 71% below the poverty line (HMG/UNICEF, 1992). Women have marginal status and gender discrimination begins in childhood. Where food is scarce, girls receive smaller amounts and poorer quality foods than their brothers. They are less likely to be immunized or to receive medical treatment when ill (Grover, 1991). Educating girls is not considered to be a priority and only 11.5% of women are literate, compared with 34.9% of men (Ali, 1991). The mean age of girls at marriage is 17.1 years, and 40% are married by 14 years of age. The total fertility rate is 5.8 children. A maternal mortality rate ranging from 515/100,000 live births in urban populations to 1600/100,000 live births in rural areas reflects the poor health status of women. Further indicators are the high neonatal mortality rates (35/1000 live births in urban areas and 150/1000 live births in rural areas) and the 29% incidence of low birth weight babies (< 2500 g) (Ali, 1991; HMG, 1992).

The Ministry of Health was officially established in 1956. Curative care became available at hospitals in urban centres, although there was no health care delivery system outside Kathmandu Valley. At this time the maternity hospital in Kathmandu, Prasuti Griha, was built.

In Western countries maternity services developed over several centuries during which women themselves were also developing politically. In Nepal, the maternity services were modelled on Western medicine and have been instituted intact, over a matter of a few decades. Women in Nepal are not aware of their rights, nor have they knowledge of the means and political structures through which to make their voices heard (HMG/UNICEF, 1992).

THE NEED FOR WOMAN-ORIENTATED RESEARCH

Literature on Nepali women's views of maternity services is scarce or inaccessible, and the available literature tends to focus on traditional practices. This reflects a general lack of literature on women's views of formal maternity services in developing countries. This is partly related to women's marginal status, but also to three assumptions that underlie health development programmes. The first is that international (Western or Western-trained) medical experts know best the type of care appropriate for child-bearing women. The second is that the medical model of maternity care is universally appropriate. The third is that illiterate or minimally educated women with little social, economic, or political power are incapable of setting priorities for their own care in child-bearing (Brems and Griffiths, 1992).

Little has changed since Campbell et al. (1979) stated that: "In Nepal social science research for development is presently dominated by the questionnaire survey method." They found that data gathered by these surveys were often incorrect due to inappropriate, cross-cultural use of research instruments. They concluded that in order to improve internal validity, research in developing countries requires a combination of methods, including in-depth interviews and participant observation.

The study presented here is about child-bearing as defined by the women themselves. Critical ethnography was the methodology used. An important quality of social science research in general, and ethnography in particular, is reflexivity. This is the recognition that the researcher is part of the social world being studied and alters a situation by being present. It also acknowledges that social scientists do not observe a static and 'objective' reality. The 'reality' being investigated is constantly undergoing change according to the meanings and interpretations given to events by the participants, and their responses to these.

THE STUDY OF WOMEN'S EXPERIENCES OF HOSPITAL BIRTH IN KATHMANDU

Field work was carried out in the public maternity ward of Prasuti Griha maternity hospital over a 3-month period. The hospital serves the Kathmandu Valley population of about 700,000, and in 1994 had about 15,000 obstetric admissions. The study questions were:

- Who are the women who come to the hospital to have their first baby?
- What do they do?
- What do they want?
- What do they need?

Depth interviews were conducted with 30 women, all first-time mothers with no history of antenatal in-patient care. They had all experienced a spontaneous onset of labour and had given birth without complication to a 'normal' baby. Low birth weight infants were included because of the high incidence of low birth weight in the hospital (28%), and because special management is only followed in exceptional cases. These mothers and babies had been 'discharged' from the hospital and were selected from the hospital record book.

The mothers were conversant in Nepali, the language in which the interviews were conducted. Each woman gave permission to have the interview tape recorded. Personal names and demographic information were not taped, but were recorded in a field notebook. Women were invited to tell their own story from the time of becoming pregnant. A set of open-ended questions were used as prompts, although discussion was not restricted to these. A young Nepali woman assisted in the interviews. She had been born in a remote village and was similar in age to the mothers.

The first five interviews were carried out in the home, with four of these women interviewed again after 2 months. The other 25 interviews were carried out on the postnatal ward. The behaviour of the mothers being interviewed, other mothers on the ward, and staff routines, attitudes, and practices were observed during the interview period. After completion of the interviews a series of visits were made to the antenatal and labour wards to gather information through observation and discussions with staff members. Hospital notes and patient records were referred to infrequently.

Women's accounts of their experiences were documented and analysis conducted for the socio-cultural and medical service implications relating to access to care, appropriate care, and quality of care. The three accounts given here (see boxes on pages 104–106) reveal issues which recurred throughout the experiences of the 30 women interviewed.

USE OF MATERNITY SERVICES

Although all the mothers interviewed gave birth in hospital, access to health care was still an issue. Their use of services was examined in order to understand their expectations and requirements of maternity services.

Like Sushila (see box on page 104), more than a third of women interviewed did not attend the antenatal clinic. Some attended only once, to register or "to see if the baby was all right." Fewer than half attended more than once. Some, like Kamala (see box on page 105), went because they felt unwell. Others were part of an extended family in the city and considered it 'modern' to use the hospital services.

Sushila

Sushila is a 17-year-old Newar. She was married at age 15^1/$_2$. She and her husband left their village 6 months ago and came to find work in Kathmandu. She was pregnant. Neither has been to school and neither is literate.

They rent a room in a run down clay-brick building which houses several other households, each in one room. Sushila's husband works as a labourer from six in the morning to six at night. Since the baby was born, he has been cooking their *daal bhaat* (lentil soup, white rice, and a curried vegetable, usually potato), morning and evening. Sushila says the other women also help. They live 5 minutes' walk from a private clinic and about 15 minutes from the Maternity Hospital.

"I did not go for any care in pregnancy. I had no problems. When the pains came I stayed at home for 1 day. I expected having a baby would be hard. Then my husband and I went to the hospital. It took 3 days for the baby to come (a boy, 3.10 kg). My husband was not allowed to stay with me; he had to wait outside. Having the baby was easy, but the labour pains were long. They gave the baby to me right away and I fed it. The nurses did not explain anything to me and they are mean.

"I would tell a friend to go to hospital for the delivery. It would be difficult to have a baby at home. To have the baby would be OK, but the placenta is attached to the baby and it can be hard to get out. I would tell a friend, it will be all right in the end."

At a home visit 2 months later, the baby looked fat and healthy; Sushila looked thin and wan. The baby had been immunized at the hospital clinic '45 days after birth'. Sushila knows that the immunizations are to prevent diseases.

"I don't want another baby soon. Maybe in 5 years. I will go for an injection after my first period comes. I heard that on the radio, maybe; I'm not sure. But the injections are available in medical shops and at the hospital clinic. I'm going to start giving the baby bottle milk. It wants to feed 2 or 3 hours after its last feed. My milk is not enough."

Sushila and her husband are looking for a cheaper room to live in. They cannot afford the one they have.

A hospital delivery was planned by only about half of the women. As one woman said, "In the village there is your mother-in-law and other people to look after you. But here there is nobody to help." Three women who had registered at the antenatal clinic would have preferred to stay at home for delivery, but at some point in the labour came to hospital because "the baby was not coming nicely at home." Others, who had never attended the clinic, took a 'wait and see' attitude, and ended up going spontaneously because of anxiety or advice from someone.

During labour and delivery, companions "had to stay outside." Husbands were given a written order for "saline and injections" that they were required to buy at the hospital medical shop. The women said "saline was given, and injections to make pain." For delivery they were taken to the delivery room, except a few like Kamala, whose babies came in the antenatal bed. They were "cut and sewn below" and told "everybody having a first baby is cut." Some mothers were grateful for this. "I couldn't stand any more, so the nurse did this and that and got the baby out." But others had

Kamala

Kamala is from a Sherpa village in an eastern hill area. Three years ago, at age 15, she came to the city to find work. She met Chhabi, a cutter, at the carpet factory where she is a weaver. They were married last year. Kamala has never been to school, but her husband has his School Leaving Certificate. They live in a room below the carpet factory. Many other men, women, and children live there also and they share a communal meal of *daal bhaat*, morning and evening.

"When I was 5 months pregnant I got swollen. Everywhere. And my stomach was big and I had pain in my liver. So I went to the hospital clinic and I went to my appointments until I was more than 8 months (the hospital is about an hour away by buses or 20 minutes by taxi, but the taxi costs a day's pay). They told me I should come to the hospital to have the baby because I was swollen and big. When labour pains started my husband took me to the hospital. In about 3 hours a baby came quickly in the waiting bed, not the delivery bed, and the nurse put her hand on my stomach and said there was another. Nobody knew there were two! I was given the babies right away and I fed them. We came home the next day."

At the time of the interview at home (in their room), a couple of days after the babies were born, there was an uncovered bottle with a couple of millilitres of milk in it sitting on the window ledge, and a tin of milk powder on a shelf. Kamala said both babies breastfed well, but that probably her milk wasn't enough for two, so they were giving powdered milk also, and someone else could feed the babies while she worked upstairs in the factory.

Another home visit was made 2 months later. The babies had not been taken for immunization. The hospital was far and it meant time off work and fare for transport. Kamala does not know what the immunizations are for. Chhabi knows they are to prevent disease. The babies were being fed by both breast and bottle. They appeared healthy, although one was noticeably smaller than the other, and quieter. Kamala and Chhabi say they make sure both babies get fed fairly.

Kamala did not know that there was a family planning clinic at the maternity hospital. She said, "Nobody here (at the factory) uses family planning. I don't want to be pregnant again for 5 years because we have two. But I don't know what to do. We know of a woman who died after taking the injections for 5 years, and another is using Norplant and is getting very thin and is going to die. I have to work hard weaving and the capsules might move to another place in my body. I'm afraid to use family planning."

When she has another baby, if she feels fine, she will not use the hospital services. She will stay at home.

quite a different experience. Sushila referred to the staff as "mean". Another uneducated, village-born young mother said, "The nurses shout. They don't help, and oh, the terrible things they do to get the baby out!" Luxmi (see box on page 106), also found the nurses harsh.

Opinions about care providers were classified into 'good', 'OK', 'not good/mean', and 'no comment'; the mothers' opinions were distributed equally across all these

Luxmi

Luxmi and her husband were both born in Kathmandu and are Newar. Luxmi is 26 years old and was married a year ago. She and her husband are tailors and both finished grade eight at school. They live according to tradition, in his extended family home, but without his mother, who had died.

"From the second month of pregnancy I went regularly to the clinic at Paton Hospital (missionary hospital), which is closer than Prasuti Griha. I knew the baby was coming when I had pains and then the waters came. After a few hours I couldn't stand it any more, so I came to the hospital. My husband and I agreed. Everybody agreed. No one else has had their baby in hospital; I am the first in the family. At the hospital the nurse wrote three kinds of medicine that we had to buy. They gave me saline. We came to the hospital at 12 o'clock, the baby was born at one thirty. The baby is fine, feeding fine. My wound hurts.

I think whether someone comes to hospital or not is their own decision. I would advise hospital. At home there would be no one to give care. At home if we cannot deliver the baby we may die. At the hospital the doctor will help. Of the two at least one will survive. At home both may die. The staff are harsh. Babies come slowly, but they try and take it out fast. It hurts us a lot. We scream a lot, but that is normal. They shout at us. They shouldn't do that. It's like that for everyone, isn't it? It would be the same for them. For everybody it is like that, everybody's body is the same. But they don't think about that. I would say to the doctors and nurses, "You should talk respectfully. You should be loving".

categories. Statements included, "Some are good. Some are bad", "They said nothing. I said nothing", "It's OK. They come to see if you are all right and they feed you." Very few of the women said they had been assisted with baby care or breastfeeding. They did not indicate these to be expectations. When asked specifically about information received, all but a few said no one had explained anything. The advice received by some was, "wash your wound with Dettol water; wash your nipples with hot water and milk will come."

Birth weights of 18 of the babies in the study group were available. Of these, 11 were low birth weight (< 2500 g). The only time mothers were aware of having a 'small baby' was if it 'went upstairs' (to the special care baby unit). When the baby was returned to the mother, nothing was said regarding the baby's needs or care.

The majority of mothers were comfortable with breastfeeding and satisfied with how the baby was doing. However, in the first 24 hours after giving birth about a fifth of them said, "Milk isn't coming." Among these, one was giving powdered milk feeds and another was planning to send her husband to buy a bottle and get milk from a nearby tea shop. Some of the women said they hurt so much from their 'wound' (episiotomy) that they could not manage breastfeeding. At a follow-up visit of four breastfeeding mothers a couple of months later, two were supplementing with artificial feeds and another was planning to do so.

When asked about a next baby, women replied: "Who knows?" Even some of those who replied, "One is enough," did not know how they could delay or avoid another pregnancy. When family planning methods or, more specifically, methods to prevent having a baby were raised, almost a half said they did not know about it. Some thought that their husband might know. About half of the women expressed interest in deferring the next pregnancy. They referred to "the injection" and Norplant. However, as with Kamala, there was a good deal of anxiety over the hazards they had heard associated with its use.

For a next delivery, half said they would not use the hospital services unless problems forced them to do so. "If it's difficult at home, go to hospital. If not, stay home." Those who were planning to use the hospital services said, "In the city you go to the hospital," or, "In the hospital the doctors and nurses can save lives."

PRIVATE LIVES AND PUBLIC SERVICES

How do the private lives of these mothers relate to the public issues of maternity services? In this study, lack of awareness of health issues, low social status, lack of a sense of control, and perceived inappropriateness of care among the mothers were evident. However, the most significant factor was culture: village culture or city culture.

In the village culture, giving birth is considered a normal event, expected to occur within a year of marriage and at intervals thereafter. It takes place within the family and the community. At every stage of the child-bearing process there are traditions to follow, and rituals to perform to win the favour of the gods and evoke their goodwill and consequent health for mother and baby. Generally, the person responsible for advice and care is the mother-in-law. Hospital services are viewed as curative. The village-born women in this study went to the hospital when they felt they had problems or needed someone to care for them. Urbanization had led to a loss of the traditional care givers and support systems available in the village.

The 'wait and see' philosophy is also encouraged, both by the fatalism inherent in Hinduism and by the great difficulty, in reality, of influencing the course of life given the conditions and resources in village life (Bista, 1991).

Being illiterate, and living in a community where there is general illiteracy among the women, prevents access to written information about health needs during child-bearing, and to the nature of the services available. Illiteracy and a village background, even more than caste, become overt stigma in hospital. "Uneducated. Thirteen, fourteen years old; it's these village girls from the factories that give us all the trouble! They think having a baby is normal!" said an obstetrician vehemently. Attitudes implicit in this statement may further ensure that the hospital is viewed only as a place to go under the extreme threat of dying or when one is desperate for some care.

Scant economic resources also reduced the likelihood of using the health services. Why use hospital services when the many costs (transport, 'compulsory' medicines, delivery charge, daily bed charge, something to 'slip' the attendant for assistance, time away from work) can be avoided?

Women from the 'city culture', on the other hand, tended to view hospital as a place that offers preventive care. It was said that in the antenatal clinic doctors and nurses could check if the baby was all right and give tetanus injections and vitamins. During delivery, family and traditions might go unacknowledged, but lives could be saved.

The interviews revealed much about the way poor women view their lives and their futures. This information can be examined to highlight the ways in which these young women are vulnerable, and the ways in which they are strong.

WHERE THE WOMEN ARE VULNERABLE
Health status
A third of the mothers were in their teens, socially and emotionally young. Their health status was poor as a result of gender discrimination, and physical development was not yet complete (Royston and Armstrong, 1989). They were predisposed to problems in child-bearing (Grover, 1991). These women need special support and care to enhance their own growth and development, to facilitate safe childbirth, and to have healthy babies. The high number of low birth weight babies is an indication of the women's poor health overall.

Diet
Most of the women and their husbands were unskilled labourers. Working hours were long and they survived on minimal food. *Daal bhaat* is the national dish because the *daal* (lentils) and *bhaat* (white rice) are available to most of the population. There are other inexpensive foods which can be cultivated easily in small spaces (notably 'greens', beans, and peas), but awareness of nutritional content and needs is lacking.

Living arrangements and social support
These women were first-time mothers and thus inexperienced. Almost three-quarters were recently from villages, and lacked care or direction from older women of their family. They were without their friends and the support systems of village life.

Education
Half of the women had never been to school; another quarter had grade five or less; one-quarter of their husbands had never been to school and about half had high-school education. These women need information through the media and channels that do not rely on the written word. Husbands and wives need the opportunity to acquire new information together as, contrary to tradition, they were living in nuclear families.

Views on child-bearing
As we have already seen, the women from villages tended to view child-bearing as a normal family-centred event. Hospitals were a place to go when there were problems. Most of the women from the city culture felt that it was modern to receive care in hospital. None mentioned her own health in relation to antenatal care. The only available options for delivery were to have the baby at home with an untrained person, or in hospital. Half of the women in this study had no knowledge of the importance of having the care of a trained attendant. Women need access to trained attendants who will care for them on their terms. While emergency services must be available, universal hospital care is not the best way to offer support for healthy child-bearing (Richards, 1978; Tew, 1990; Sundari, 1992).

Babies
Mothers did not indicate an awareness that a low-weight baby requires special attention to protect its health, nor did they have information about the factors that contribute to having a low-weight baby. The women were generally able to care for their babies and followed the village practice of wrapping them in layers. They fed

on demand and each day rubbed the baby with oil and put it in the sun for a short time. These beneficial practices could be incorporated into a broader understanding of the needs of their babies.

Breastfeeding

There was a lack of knowledge about breastfeeding. Some women stated that their milk did not come after delivery or was insufficient. Others were supplementing with powdered milk within 2 months of delivery. Two- or three-hourly feeds were seen as a sign of insufficient milk production. In villages supplementary feeding is common. A grandmother minding a baby may give boiled buffalo milk and sugar on a spoon. None of the mothers in the study spoke about the hazards of artificial feeds. Some of the women said the pain from their episiotomy interfered with breastfeeding. The possible implication of episiotomies in difficulties with the initiation of breastfeeding merits further investigation.

Family planning

None of the mothers used contraception to delay a first birth. Traditionally, proof of being able to bear children is eagerly awaited after marriage. In villages it is important to have many children: girls to work in the home and fields; sons for religious purposes and to bring economic resources, wives, and grandchildren into the family to provide for parents in old age. A third of the women in this study indicated a desire to postpone or avoid a next pregnancy.

WHERE THE WOMEN ARE STRONG

None of the women who had left the village for the city expressed regret at their decision. They were courageous women leaving all that was familiar in the belief that they could make a better life. This is a rejection of the fatalism of Hinduism and of village thinking. It was also an action taken by the women and their husbands together. Some women, like Kamala, who lived and worked in a carpet factory, were members of a community, even if it was a relatively new community. This may have been true for other women.

Appropriate care for the women in this study would be care that is accessible in terms of the socio-cultural patterns of their lives, that meets their health needs in child-bearing, that builds on their strengths, and that does not foster dependency.

THE MATERNITY SERVICES AND ISSUES OF QUALITY OF CARE

In developing countries, quality of care and its association with the use of services has received much attention, most noticeably in the area of family planning. Donabedian (1988) stated that the relationship between patient and provider should involve, "privacy, confidentiality, informed choice, concern, empathy, honesty, tact, [and] sensitivity," since the "interpersonal process is the vehicle by which technical care is implemented and on which its success depends."

Mensch (1993) suggested four general dimensions for assessment of quality of care in relation to women's health services: provider–woman information exchange, provider competence, interpersonal relations, and mechanisms to encourage continuity of medical care. This framework has been adapted here to consider the maternity service provision in Nepal. 'Appropriate provider' has been substituted for 'provider competence' in this case, and 'health care' is referred to rather than 'medical care' (because child-bearing should not be considered an illness).

Satisfactory information exchange between care providers and the women using the services requires that the provider:

- Demonstrates an understanding of the client's background, needs, and wishes, and an understanding of child-bearing and of the services provided.
- Imparts information about processes and procedures, rationale, and options.
- Clarifies her client's understanding of these.

At Prasuti Griha an average work-load in the daily, 2-hour antenatal clinic was 80 new cases. Nurse-midwives weighed, measured blood pressure, and took a history from each woman who was a new case. All the examinations were done by doctors or medical students, male or female. More than one woman was examined in a room at a time and there was no partition between them. There was no opportunity for the mothers to meet and talk with the nurse alone. Despite the existence of a video machine, the clinic was not an environment that promoted or encouraged information exchange.

When the women arrived at the hospital in labour, they were given a prescription for 'compulsory' medicines (dextrose/saline, Syntocinon, IV tubing, syringes, and needles) to buy at the hospital pharmacy. They never understood what they were buying, or why. The routine use of Syntocinon augmentation, and of performing episiotomies on first-time mothers, was not discussed. Most of the care on the antenatal and postnatal wards was given by untrained ward attendants. Most women went home the day after delivery. On their way out they stopped at the desk of the staff nurse or auxiliary-nurse-midwife (ANM), who told them quickly and didactically the regimen for any medicines they might be using, and that they should return in 45 days to have their baby immunized. No information was given regarding low-weight babies, breastfeeding, or why immunization was needed. Family planning was not discussed.

This lack of mechanisms to encourage continuity of health care was evident in many areas. Clinic staff stated to the interviewers that in the postnatal clinic women were examined, counselled about family planning, and the baby immunized. However, this does not always seem to have happened. Of the four women in this study followed up at 2 months, only two returned to the maternity hospital to have their babies immunized. Both were considering contraception in order to postpone the next pregnancy, but neither was informed nor aware that family planning services were available in another part of the building. It was observed that women using the services were not encouraged to participate actively, but rather pressured to be compliant. Questions were considered ignorant and mocked.

Interpersonal relations were rarely considered important. Providers of care assumed that a physical examination by a doctor was necessary and sufficient. Women using the services saw the care providers as people with training who could assess the well-being of the baby *in utero*, "take a baby out", and "save women's lives". Many also assumed that poor women such as themselves were in no position to say anything about doctors and nurses, and should not expect respect.

The high turnover of patients in large hospitals is often given as justification for the lack of personal support offered. Staff in this hospital indicated that more personalized care was a luxury available only to those with the economic means to pay for it (e.g., through private rooms). Frequent references were made to too many patients, too few staff, and too little equipment. Yet, during the research visits there was overt inactivity and socializing among staff members, even while women exhibited obvious signs of needing help. It is of interest that none of the women in this study made a distinction between doctors, nurses, ANMs, and ward attendants in their accounts, perhaps because there was little difference in their attitudes towards the women from which to distinguish them.

Observation revealed frequent verbal and non-verbal reinforcement of an 'us and them' distinction between staff and 'patients'. On several occasions women crying in pain were ignored by staff. On two occasions that we observed on the postnatal ward, attendants shouted at weeping women saying, "It's normal to have pain." On another occasion, a 21-year-old mother who had two children 15 months apart in age was subjected by a nurse to a very public reprimand for having had babies so close together. Such incidents indicate that respect and honesty are not considered to be qualities required of the care providers in offering service.

An *appropriate provider* should have training, knowledge, and experience appropriate for the jobs or tasks to which she is assigned. It is useful to examine the assumptions upon which staffing was based. Several nurses and ANMs were asked whether they had a job description. They said they did not. This is consistent with the findings of an unpublished study, carried out by the Division of Nursing, of 50 nurses at various hospitals in Kathmandu (Levitt, 1993). A nursing supervisor stated, however, that job descriptions were on file somewhere.

In the antenatal and family planning clinics four of the nurses had received an extra year of training in public health, which included maternal health and child-bearing. Yet there was no opportunity for women coming to the clinic to meet with them to discuss health issues or to ask questions. All antenatal care is provided by doctors and medical students, who only look for deviations from normal in the physical parameters of pregnancy.

Every antenatal and postnatal ward was staffed by either a staff nurse or an ANM and ward attendants. Despite very different training, the staff nurse and the ANM said they were interchangeable and did the same work. The *de facto* role of the staff member on the ward was record keeping, communicating with the doctors, giving care to 'medical cases' (women with complications), and supervising the ward attendants. The ward attendants actually provided the direct patient care. Thus, most of the care of labouring women and of postnatal mothers and their babies was carried out by untrained women with a grade five education.

A Baby Friendly Initiative to support breastfeeding has been initiated at Prasuti Griha. Reports from UNICEF (Manandhar, 1993) were that all doctors (more than 50) and four nursing supervisors had attended a workshop on breastfeeding. Two nursing supervisors then ran workshops for all of their staff. A workshop was not held for the ward attendants, in spite of their current key role.

The general assumption behind staffing and job delegation appeared to be that a doctor was the appropriate primary service provider for all pregnant women. The staff actually providing most of the care for women during labour and in the immediate postnatal period were not considered to require any special knowledge or training, while trained staff were required for administration and for 'abnormal cases'.

GIVEN THE LIMITATIONS, IS QUALITY POSSIBLE?

Quality of care needs to be discussed from the perspective of the person needing or receiving care. The provision of optimal physical, social, and emotional health should be a goal in its own right, but it is also an important way of encouraging women to use the services. Standards for measuring quality do need to be established. A universal standard may not be possible given the discrepancies in facilities, economics, staffing, and other country- and location-specific factors. However, it is not unrealistic to expect "a normative standard of care – that is, a standard which is acceptable and achievable ..." (Mensch, 1993), which specifies a basic minimum standard of quality of care.

Prasuti Griha has many constraints – a limited budget, a large number of clients, and the available physical facilities, but it has the potential to provide more appropriate and better care even within these constraints. What is required is a change of attitude and perspective by the administration and staff, and some recommendations are included here.

In the longer term a change in the infrastructure and organization of care is also required, to provide outreach services in the community. Women do need emergency hospital services for emergency care. However, they also need community-based services where information and care are readily available from midwives who know 'who they are, what they do, and what they want'. They need services that support them where they are vulnerable and encourage them in their strengths.

REFERENCES

Ali, A. (1991) *Status of Health in Nepal.* Resource Centre for Primary Health Care, Nepal and South–South Solidarity, Kathmandu.

Bista, D.B. (1991) *Fatalism and Development.* Orient Longman, Calcutta.

Brems, S. and Griffiths, M. (1992) Health women's way: Learning to listen. In: Koblinsky, M., Timyan, J., and Gay, J. (eds), *The Health of Women: A Global Perspective.* Westview Press, Boulder, CA.

Campbell, J.G., Shrestha, R., and Stone, L. (1979) *The Use And Misuse of Social Science Research in Nepal.* Research Centre for Nepal and Asian Studies, Tribhwan University, Kirtipur, Kathmandu.

Chalmers, I., Enkin, M., and Keirse, M.J.N.C. (eds) (1989) *Effective Care in Pregnancy and Childbirth.* Oxford University Press, Oxford.

Donabedian, A. (1988) The quality of care: How can it be assessed? *Journal of the American Medical Association,* **260**(12): 1743–1748.

Grover, D. (1991) *Hamra Chelibetiharu: An Analysis of the Situation of the Girl Children in Nepal.* UNICEF, Kathmandu.

HMG (1992) *The Safe Motherhood Initiative in Nepal: Situation Analysis With Suggested Policies and Strategies.* Ministry of Health, Nepal. Unpublished draft.

HMG/UNICEF (1992) *Children and Women of Nepal: A Situation Analysis.* National Planning Commission, HMG Nepal and UNICEF, Kathmandu.

Levitt, (1993) Personal communication.

Manandhar, V. (1993) Personal communication. UNICEF, Kathmandu.

Mensch, B. (1993) Quality of care: A neglected dimension. In: Koblinsky, M., Timyan, J., and Gay, J. (eds), *The Health of Women: A Global Perspective*. Westview Press, Boulder, CA.

Richards, M.P.M. (1978) A place of safety? An examination of the risks of hospital delivery. In: Kitzinger, S. and Davis, J.K. (eds), *The Place of Birth*. Oxford University Press, Oxford.

Royston, E. and Armstrong, S. (eds) (1989) *Preventing Maternal Deaths*. WHO, Geneva.

Sundari, T.K. (1992) The untold story: How the health care systems in developing countries contribute to maternal mortality. *National Journal of Health Services*, **22**(3), pp 513–528.

Tew, M. (1990) *Safer Childbirth?* Chapman & Hall, London.

Recommendations for Prasuti Griha Maternity Hospital

A POLICY OF WOMEN-CENTRED CARE

- *Midwife (ANM) as primary provider.* The care of the normal child-bearing woman is her professional mandate and, "the practice should be abandoned of involving doctors or obstetricians in the care of every pregnant woman" (Chalmers et al., 1989).
- *Active participation by women in their own care.* Including options such as choosing not to have unnecessary interventions, to be mobile during labour, to have a female attendant for delivery, and the position for delivery.
- *Recognition of women's social and emotional needs.* Including labour support from a friend or family member, respect, privacy during examinations, confidentiality.
- Supportive, non-interventionist care for normal childbirth, according to recommendations of recent research (Chalmers et al., 1989).
- Provision of relevant information and education in a manner appropriate to a woman's background and needs.

STAFF DEVELOPMENT

- A job description agreed upon by staff members and hospital.
- Education, training, and experience appropriate to the individual's assignment.
- Training for all staff who give direct care. Ward attendants providing care require knowledge about women's needs in labour, breastfeeding, dangers of bottle feeds, care of low-weight babies, immunization, and family planning.
- Accountability to a senior staff member.

Protocols and procedure guidelines for each clinical area

- Criteria for basic minimum standards of care and of practice that are acceptable, achievable, and can be monitored effectively.
- Monitoring tools by which to assess adherence to standards of practice and procedure guidelines.
- Review of the use and accessibility of facilities.

Improving Quality of Care for Women: The Story of the *Casa del Parto*, Nicaragua

Ramona Alfaro Morales

This is the story of one innovative health project in the north of Nicaragua, designed and run by nurses and midwives, which set out to improve the standard of maternity care available to women within both the formal health services and the informal sector.

THE CONTEXT

Before the success of the Sandinista revolution, Nicaragua had been ruled by the wealthy Somoza family. Little of that wealth was shared. The poor health of the general population was clearly indicated by high infant mortality rates. In some regions of the country, these figures reached 120/1000 live births (CELADE, 1988). Fertility rates were high and life expectancy was 50 years. Some of the main causes of death were due to poor living conditions (diarrhoea, malnutrition, parasitaemia, tuberculosis). Many deaths were preventable by vaccination, such as measles, poliomyelitis, and tetanus. Although national statistics for the period are unreliable, it is clear that maternal and perinatal deaths caused by limited access to emergency health services were common.

Within this morbidity and mortality profile, there were acute differences between rural and urban populations. The Somoza regime devoted few resources to solving health problems. What was available went to the main urban bases of the country, with a dynamic in which charity and commerce rubbed shoulders, and privileges were granted to curative services. Large sectors of the population were excluded from health care, especially those in rural areas. They had to solve their problems by buying drugs without prescription, and by using the informal systems of health care available among the population. Less than 15% of births occurred in public health facilities. A small minority gave birth as paying clients in private hospitals and clinics, and the rest remained in the care of uncertified traditional midwives, the *parteras*.

When social tensions increased, in the final years of the dictatorship, some public health programmes, such as latrine building and provision of birth control, were carried out in association with community programmes, but these had clear political objectives in that they focused on those municipalities in which opposition to the regime was developing.

In 1979 the revolution succeeded in removing the dictatorship. The immediate health situation worsened as there were hundreds of dead and injured, and massive destruction of service infrastructures caused by the armed forces of the outgoing regime. There were also indirect effects caused by the paralysis of production and agriculture during the last months of the dictatorship, followed by decapitalization carried out by the associates of the former government.

Once this tempestuous period had passed, finding an answer to the most urgent health problems of the population became imperative. Redistribution of the available resources to meet the needs of the whole population began with the creation of the Sistema Nacional Unico de Salud (National Health Service). One of the first tasks was the organization of the Departmental Health Offices, commissioned to reactivate health services, and to guarantee health care to all, including the rural population.

This meant that the pre-existing services would now have to provide for a far greater population base than before. The strain on the services was compounded by the exodus of many professionals to Miami, following their better-off clients. It was necessary to create extra nursing schools, mainly to prepare auxiliary nursing personnel, and to send large numbers of students to several National Institutions in order to pursue health related studies. Much of this training was funded through international aid and solidarity.

With the establishment of regional health authorities, a process of decentralization of resources began and, at the same time, close relationships were established with community organizations. At a primary care level, outreach maternal and child health (MCH) programmes were developed and extended throughout the country, emphasizing the management of oral rehydration, antenatal care, vaccinations, health education for the population, programmes for children under 6 years of age (growth and development control), and so on. The massive health education programme was based on the training of community agents (members of health brigades from communities and work places, and the traditional midwives), and these ultimately became very important elements in health development. Concurrent revitalization of the economy, the national crusade for literacy, and developments in the state education services made possible a major improvement in the health situation.

In the years 1984–1987, this advancing process was interrupted violently by the increase in low-intensity warfare conducted by the *contra*, groups of mercenaries and supporters of the ex-dictator. The attacks hampered the development of the national health project, most acutely of all in the northern region, and much energy had to be diverted towards defence.

The war forced modifications in health care activities. Health personnel in the war zones could no longer move about freely to do outreach work, and had to curtail their health promotion activities in rural areas, abandoning some health posts when these became the focus of armed attack. The continuing vaccination campaigns were carried out at great personal risk to health service personnel, as government workers were considered legitimate targets for kidnap and torture by the *contra*. Influxes of internal refugees provoked further demand for urban units. The available hospital beds could not be used fully because they needed to be ready for emergencies due to military actions. Surgical services became a priority for the same reason, in spite of other existing health problems.

During this period the development of health services stagnated. This was reflected in a deterioration in the health status indicators, with an increase in morbidity and mortality. In 15–49-year-olds, battle wounds became the primary cause of death.

ORIGINS OF THE *CASA REGIONAL DE PREPARACIÓN PARA EL PARTO NATURAL*

It was in this difficult context that nurses and nurse midwives were attempting to provide maternity care to the women of the region. They could see from their contact with the communities that there were many problems. Many women expressed fear of pregnancy and delivery. Maternal mortality rates did not seem to be decreasing, in spite of efforts to improve health care. There was known to be a high perinatal mortality rate, and many neonatal deaths resulted from tetanus in rural areas. There was a high incidence of home deliveries, even in urban centres. These home births were attended by *parteras*, midwives without formal training who had traditionally accompanied women through their labour and delivery, but who had no training in how to identify or deal with complications.

Care in the health facilities was basic, although it had improved a little and was now free to all. There was little knowledge among health staff about how to assist women in coping with labour. Women did not like to go to hospitals to give birth because they did not find the necessary human warmth in the delivery units of these facilities. They reported mistreatment by health professionals. They also complained of feeling isolated in a delivery room tended by unknown people. There was great fear of episiotomy. On top of all this, beds were scarce in hospitals, which sometimes made it necessary for two women to share the same bed. It was for these reasons that many preferred to stay at home with the *partera*.

Aware of this situation, and using the experience of international colleagues who were co-operating with us, a group of nurses and midwives decided to initiate some specific health activities around the problems we could see. Meetings were organized in co-ordination with the Regional Mother and Health Care (MCH) Programme to consolidate ideas and to use those experiences gained in other countries. Teaching materials, booklets, handbills, posters, and signs were designed with the aid of the MCH Programme. Several funding proposals were written for international organizations to provide economic resources, which were not available nationally. By the end of 1985, we were able to offer qualified antenatal care, preparation for childbirth for pregnant women attending for antenatal care, training programmes and follow-up for traditional midwives, and ongoing training for nursing personnel working in maternal and child health.

Since such activity was totally new in our country, our experience was very limited. We drew on the help of experienced personnel from Puerto Rico and the United States. They provided training not only to our co-ordinating team, but also to other staff from different hospitals in the region, from Somoto, La Trinidad, Estelí, and Ocotal.

The co-ordinating group of nurses and midwives also decided to try to raise funds to purchase accommodation for the educational projects. We wanted a drop-in centre where pregnant and non-pregnant women could comfortably come to obtain information about their bodies and their health from professionals, but in an environment of mutual confidence, away from any health facility. This building could also function as the base from which the training of *parteras* and health staff could be conducted. It would be a centre that would provide education and training to all those concerned with childbirth.

In October 1985 our funding application was approved by a British organization called Christian Aid, who provided the funding for the purchase of a house in Estelí (the *Casa*), which would serve as a pilot project. The co-ordinating team and the Regional MCH Programme, appointed three nurse-midwives to run the *Casa*, with support provided by the rest of the nurses who continued with their work in their own municipalities. The Ministry of Health paid the salaries of the *Casa*'s workers, and Christian Aid provided funds for equipment and programme expenses.

Thus, on 26th May 1986, the *Casa del Parto* (the house of birth, as it was locally known) in Estelí opened its doors. Its general aim was to contribute to a reduction of the maternal and infant morbidity and mortality rates of the region.

Its specific goals were:

- To provide women (and their partners) with the psychological and physical preparation necessary for childbirth without fear.
- To improve the quality of care in home delivery by providing education to traditional midwives.
- To improve the quality of maternity care provided at the government health facilities, by organizing seminars and in-service training on related subjects for health care professionals.
- To improve the reproductive health of women by providing family advice and sex education to individuals, community groups, and schools.

IMPROVING STANDARDS OF CARE IN THE INSTITUTIONS

The *Casa del Parto* has worked for nearly a decade to improve the standard of care in health centres and in the maternity unit of the regional referral hospital. Some of its staff work part time in the hospital's labour unit, where they have campaigned strenuously for the right of women to have a chosen companion in labour, to be active and mobile in labour, and to have a choice in such matters as positions for delivery and episiotomy. In 1988 the *Casa* also conducted a small observational research project within the hospital in order to highlight the inadequacies of the standards of care (Alfaro *et al.*, 1988). It has provided regional training for maternity staff in the use of the partograph and in active birth techniques, and it has provided updates in antenatal care.

PROMOTING ACTIVE BIRTH

The *Casa* has been the prime advocate of natural or active birth preparation within the country. The antenatal sessions were originally based on the Lamaze method of psychoprophylaxis, but they have been modified gradually to a more flexible active birth perspective (Casa Regional de Preparación, 1989). The preparation emphasizes an understanding of how the body works and helps women (and their chosen partners) to learn how to assist the process of pregnancy and birth with confidence and without fear. We have found that our most important task has been in helping women to overcome their inherited fear of childbirth – fear of pain, fear of losing the baby, fear of dying – and in helping them to believe that childbirth can be a powerful and a joyful experience. It is a rewarding and exhilarating task.

TRAINING FOR TRADITIONAL MIDWIVES

In Nicaragua today, still less than half of all births, about 45%, take place in institutions with the attention of health service staff or private doctors. The rest occur at home. Some mothers deliver their babies themselves, others with the help of their husband, and others, probably around 80% of the home births, are assisted by a *partera*. Even in a town like Estelí, where there is a regional hospital within relatively easy walking distance of most neighbourhoods, only 36% of women choose to give birth there (Murray, 1988). They continue to have more confidence in their traditional midwives than in the impersonal and at times unfeeling treatment in the hospital. The *partera* belongs to the community, already knows the family well, and shares the same system of beliefs about health and illness. She is either paid in kind or charges very little. She often provides antenatal massage – *sobadura* – and sometimes postnatal care (Luiser, 1985).

In the initial post-revolution period, the Sandinista government aimed not only at providing a free national health service to all citizens, but placed much emphasis on the training of doctors and on the desirability of institutional birth. Then, during the 1980s as resources were diverted into defence, community health workers and traditional midwives began to be seen as a realistic means of distributing health care to the majority of people at low cost. There was also a renewed interest in traditional healing, massage, and herbal remedies, all part of local culture.

Nicaragua became one of a number of countries which, with UNICEF backing, instituted training programmes for traditional birth attendants (TBAs) in an attempt to 'upgrade' their practice, on the assumption that this would improve maternal and child health. The estimates for the number of *parteras* in the country range from 6000 to 15,000 (Veraguas, 1988). Around 3000 have received some sort of training from Ministry of Health personnel. One survey conducted in 1987 (Ministerio de Salud, 1987) described the typical *partera* as an older woman, average age 53 years, with more than 20 years' experience, attending perhaps two or three births per month (some, of course, attend many more, and many attend much less). Of the sample, 72% were illiterate. Half of these midwives had learned their skills by attending their own births; 27% had learned from apprenticeship to another *partera*. The *partera* in Nicaragua, as in many other countries, does not exist only in the countryside. In the rapidly growing neighbourhoods on the edges of town, the *parteras* are often vital links with vulnerable women not in contact with antenatal care services.

Training these empirical midwives is not simple. The staff of the *Casa* use popular education methods that engage the *parteras* actively in the subject they are discussing. Wherever possible the language used is the language of the *parteras*, and if a medical term is used it is explained in non-medical terms also. Before the training sessions, the training team spend several days in the outlying areas working with the local health-post staff on this issue, giving them the basics of the kind of participative education methods that they need to use, and the opportunity to explore some of the different concepts and notions they might encounter. In the early days, many *parteras* came to the training courses hoping to "learn to inject," and much time was spent trying to convince them that supportiveness, clean non-interventionist practices, and the early detection of problems were far more useful and important skills.

As well as encouraging an interaction with the health centres or posts, the *Casa* actively encouraged *parteras* to bring women with problems to the hospital themselves. It argued that the *partera* should be welcomed by the hospital staff and encouraged to stay to give support to her client and to follow her case through. Sometimes this worked well, and certainly over the years *partera* referrals increased in number, but many doctors still regard the *parteras* as superstitious, ignorant, and dangerous.

The essential requirement is for good long-term follow-up to the initial training sessions. In areas where transport was not too difficult, and when the war did not disrupt communication, regular monthly follow-up meetings were held and well-attended. They gave the opportunity to discuss problems, share experiences, and collect supplies. Over time, the *parteras* developed a sense of group identity to the extent that, when the Sandinista government lost the national elections in 1990, the *parteras* united to form a regional Association of Trained *Parteras*, with the expressed aim of defending their interests, their rights to training, and continued resources and support.

EXPANSION OF *CASA*'S ROLE

During the course of time, this centre has broadened its activities, moving with the changing circumstances and increased awareness of the problems that affect women. In the initial period, the work of the *Casa* was largely educational and much of it was on the preparation of teaching materials, information booklets using cartoon strips, and filming videos with local people. As well as the work around improving maternity care, staff were invited increasingly to give talks in schools, women's groups, work places, and co-operatives on issues related to sex education and family planning.

Programmes for the provision of antenatal care and cervical screening at the centre were introduced in subsequent years. The incidence of cervical cancer appears to be rising in Nicaragua, and routine screening facilities have often been inadequate at the health centres, so we have incorporated this into our work. The slides are sent to the pathology department at the hospital, and we receive the results and counsel those who require treatment.

THE *ALBERGUE*

In 1991 a study was carried out to estimate the maternal mortality rate in Region One by using the 'sisterhood method' in a community-based household survey. The results showed a rate eight times greater than the previous Ministry of Health estimates, with 243 deaths per 100,000 live births. Of these deaths, 60% occur at home. The lifetime risk of maternal death was calculated at 0.145 (1 in 69) (Danel, 1993). Staff from the *Casa* assisted in this survey, and when we learnt the results we decided to take further action that focused on the needs of rural women. We decided to expand the function of the *Casa del Parto* to become *un Albergue*, a maternity waiting home for women from rural areas who had been identified as being at high obstetric risk. These women can be referred to us by health service staff or by the *parteras*, or, indeed, can self-refer if they feel that they have a problem. This flexibility in accepting referrals from outside the formal health sector is an important feature. It reduces delay and it acknowledges both the *partera*'s role in the community and women's right to have a say in where they seek their care.

In March 1994 the *Albergue* opened, and in the first 9 months we received 103 women from the more isolated areas of the department of Estelí. Of these, 10% had breech presentations, 10% were teenagers (aged 15 years or younger) with their first pregnancies, and 20% were grand multiparous women with eight or more pregnancies. We have learnt much through having these women living with us at the *Casa* for 2 or 3 weeks and exchanging experiences. These conversations led us to the conclusion that we are not doing enough if we simply attend to the risk of the current pregnancy. Many of these women need to be able to prevent, or plan, subsequent pregnancies. To help them the *Casa* needs to offer a complete family planning programme, with a range of methods and counselling on the advantages and disadvantages of each, so that the women can choose their preference in an informed manner.

We have set up a service to provide oral contraceptives, intrauterine contraceptive devices (IUCDs), condoms, and surgical sterilization for women. Initially, we provided this only to the postnatal women of the maternity waiting home (of whom 68% take up the offer of contraception, 40% request sterilization, and 28% IUCD), but today we also make the service available to the population of the town. The supplies come from the Ministry of Health, as does the doctor who performs the sterilizations.

It has not all been as easy as it may sound. We have had some difficulties, mainly financial, with the running of the waiting home. Christian Aid helped us with the costs of expanding our work, but the Ministry of Health does not supply us with a budget with which to feed the women who come to the waiting home, even though it is its responsibility to do so. We still do not have a vehicle to transport women to hospital when they go into labour; we have to walk with them, or beg a neighbour for the loan of a vehicle if they cannot walk. We are still waiting to get a telephone so as to be able to call for an ambulance in case of an emergency. Lack of resources means that we have to charge women 25.00 cordobas (US$ 3.75) for sterilization by MINILAP and 5.00 cordobas for the cervical smear. Previously, this service had been free to the population, but we are so short of materials that we have to cover some costs.

Our project was born in difficult times, and has survived more than one crisis. Today our team consists of five Nicaraguan nurses and nurse-midwives, and one Swedish midwife. The *Casa del Parto* is now devoted to the integrated reproductive health care of women, combining educational and clinical services which accord women a dignified and active role.

REFERENCES

Alfaro, R., Boyle, D., Thomas, L. *et al.* (1988) *Investigación de la atención del parto en relación a la normativa del MINSA en el hospital Alejandro Davila Bolaños.* Estelí, Nicaragua. Unpublished.

Casa Regional de Preparación para el Parto Natural, (1989) Guía Práctica para Realizar la Preparación para el Parto Natural. Estelí, Nicaragua. (mimeo)

CELADE (1988) *La mortalidad en la niñez en Centroamerica, Panama y Belice: Nicaragua 1970–1986.* CELADE, San José.

Danel, I. (1993) *Estimación de la magnitude de la mortalidad materna en la Región 1 de Nicaragua usando el método de supervivencia de hermanas.* Maternal and Child Epidemiology Unit (MCEU), London School of Hygiene and Tropical Medicine, London. Unpublished report.

Luisier, V. (1985) *Te voy a ayudar nada más. Apuntes sobre las parteras empíricas en Nicaragua.* MINSA, Managua.

Ministerio de Salud (1987) *Documento Central, Primero Congreso Regional de Parteras Adiestradas Región 1.* MINSA, Nicaragua.

Murray, S.F. (1988) Unpublished report to Catholic Institute for International Relations, Canonbury Yard, 190a New North Road, London N1, UK (Region 1 Ministry of Health figures).

Veraguas, S. (1988) Unpublished report to the Catholic Institute for International Relations, Canonbury Yard, 190a New North Road, London N1, UK.

Women Organize Their Own Health Care: A Case Study from the Philippines

Diana G. Smith and **Sylvia Estrada-Claudio**

INTRODUCTION

The women's movement in the Philippines

In the Philippines, it is women's organizations which are making the biggest contribution to thinking around women's health, and to the need for changes in maternity services. There is a large and sophisticated women's movement in the Philippines, and many of the groups are involved in aspects of health. Most address the issue of health from a social as well as a biological perspective, and most aim to promote women's reproductive rights. Many groups are convinced that the present approach to the provision of medical services is not meeting the needs of the majority of women. This chapter describes some of the work of Gabriela, a coalition of women's groups, in the development of appropriate and accessible care for women.

Health problems in the Philippines

There is little doubt that the social conditions in which people in the Philippines live are having a serious adverse effect on their health. Currently, only one in four of the population has a water supply available directly or within 250 m of where they live and 30% do not have access to sanitary toilet facilities, and UNICEF estimate that the infant mortality rate is about 51.6/1000 live births (UNICEF, 1991). Protein-energy malnutrition and anaemia are common problems, particularly among young children, and pregnant and lactating women (Bongga, 1992).

Many of the leading causes of health problems faced by women and by men are both communicable and preventable. Bronchitis, influenza, diarrhoeal diseases, pneumonia, and tuberculosis topped the list in Department of Health figures for 1989 (Department of Health, 1989). Leading causes of death in women in the age group

20–24 years include diseases of the heart, tuberculosis, pneumonia, neoplasms, and accidents. The incidence of non-communicable diseases is often higher among the poorer sectors of the community, indicating a relationship with living conditions (Estrada-Claudio, 1992).

Women's health may be compromised by long hours of work and by the fact that their nutritional needs are often considered to be the lowest priority within the family. Many women face the threat of violence, either in the home or in the community.

Women's access to health services

Most of the available funding for health expenditure in the Philippines, as elsewhere, goes into city hospitals and institutions. Community services for either the rural population or the urban poor receive little funding. Much of the population lives in rural areas far from institutions that provide maternity care. The National Safe Motherhood Survey (SMS) revealed that 85% of rural deliveries took place in the home, compared with an overall figure of 70%. Of all home deliveries that occur in the Philippines, 73% are attended by a traditional birth attendant (TBA), known locally as a *hilot* (SMS, 1993).

Worryingly, the number of births delivered by *hilots* appears to have increased during recent years. Whereas in 1982 39% of all births were delivered by *hilots*, according to the Philippine Department of Health Statistics by 1986 the figure had increased to 43%. The increase in Metro Manila (the capital city) during the 1980s was particularly disturbing. In 1982, only 3.8% of births had been delivered by *hilots*, but by 1986 the rate had more than doubled to 8.4%. Apparently, the high cost of obstetricians and confinements in maternity wards was forcing more women to resort to *hilots* (Tan, 1989).

Maternal mortality

Women's groups have made particular efforts to draw attention to the high rates of maternal mortality and morbidity in the Philippines. The 1993 National Safe Motherhood Survey findings recorded a maternal mortality rate of 209 deaths per 100,000 live births (SMS, 1993).

Most maternal deaths in the Philippines are the result of hypertensive diseases, haemorrhage, and infections, many of which are preventable with better maternity care. Some of the deaths due to haemorrhage and infection may occur because of complications following unsafe, induced abortion. Abortion is illegal in the Philippines and many women are forced to use 'backstreet' services.

Pregnancy represents the fifth most likely cause of death among women in the age group 25–39 years. The death rate among very young women is a particular concern. In 1989, while there were 307 live births registered to mothers below the age of 15 years, 233 young women within that age group died of pregnancy-related complications. Statistics from previous years were similar (Tan, 1992).

For every maternal death, there are many more instances of women who suffer serious health problems that result directly from pregnancy and childbirth. Findings presented at the National Conference on Safe Motherhood in Manila in 1987 showed that the urban-poor mothers considered themselves to be in poor health generally. Over 39% of the women interviewed described problems during their most recent delivery, with 16% reporting profuse bleeding. Nearly half the women had experienced problems after delivery, with 20% reporting painful urination, and 14% reporting fever (Raymundo, 1987).

Reproductive rights

Some maternal deaths and health problems related to pregnancy could be prevented if women had the opportunity to control their fertility. In the Philippines, it has been more difficult for women to practise family planning than elsewhere in the region. Whereas there was a contraceptive prevalence of 66% in Thailand and 48% in Indonesia in the period 1983–1993, only 36% of married couples in the reproductive age group in the Philippines were using modern contraceptive methods during the same period (UNICEF, 1994).

Unlike the rest of Asia, the Philippines is a predominantly Catholic country following a 300-year history of Spanish colonial rule. The Roman Catholic Church has affected not only the services provided, but also attitudes towards modern contraceptives. Its influence and power has been particularly apparent since the opening up of public debate on issues such as family planning and abortion after the fall of the Marcos regime in 1986.

When the 'snap revolution' brought President Corazon Aquino to power, but before the new legislature was even in place, the Roman Catholic Church hierarchy, in conjunction with others, managed an intense and well-organized campaign for the inclusion of an article in the draft constitution that would protect the life of the unborn child (Dixon-Mueller and Germain, 1994). Women's groups were forced to respond by building public opposition to the draft constitution. Ultimately, it was not possible to block the clause entirely, but a clause to give equal protection to the mother was also inserted.

A second major struggle took place after the Roman Catholic Church drafted an executive order for President Aquino's signature which would have abolished POPCOM, the population commission. Many women's organizations had voiced serious doubts about some of the more coercive activities of the family planning services in the past, but they were clear that the virtual abolition of the service posed a real threat to the right to family planning and to women's health. An intense campaign by women activists, population and health professionals, and members of the public eventually resulted in the petition remaining unsigned.

Reproductive rights and health

Between 1986, when the Marcos regime fell, and 1988 the percentage of married women of reproductive age using contraceptives dropped from 45% to 36%. Observers believe that this decline in contraceptive use was the result of the pressure exerted on the Philippine government's family planning programme in that period. The long-term consequences for women's health are yet to emerge (Tan, 1992).

What is clear is that two groups of women tend to be particularly vulnerable when family planning services are reduced or restricted. One group comprises women over the age of 40 years who have often had many children with only short intervals between the births of each child. It is alarming to note that between 1986 and 1989 pregnancy-related deaths in women over 40 years of age increased (Tan, 1992). The other vulnerable group is young women. In 1989, a joint agreement signed by the government of the Philippines and the Roman Catholic Church limited contraceptive services to married couples only. It is estimated that there are currently between 720,000 and 1.32 million unmarried, female adolescents in the Philippines who are in urgent need of contraceptive advice and services (Tan, 1992).

When women's reproductive rights are restricted, there may be more abortions as a result of unwanted pregnancies. In the Philippines, abortion is illegal and therefore dangerous. According to the 1993 Safe Motherhood Survey (SMS, 1993), 24% of respondents reported having had an unwanted pregnancy, and one in five of these had taken action to end the pregnancy. Of those taking action, 5% had to be hospitalized afterwards (SMS, 1993). Various studies have revealed that 13–37% of women have attempted to have an abortion at least once. Most women who seek or undergo abortions are married, and do so after the third or fourth child (Miralao and Engracia, 1989). This finding suggests that there is an 'unmet need' for family planning services. Most women's groups in the Philippines believe that women should have the right to family planning as part of reproductive health services.

GABRIELA

Gabriela is one of the largest women's organizations in the Philippines. It is a nation-wide coalition of women's groups comprising 45,000 members. The 'Gabriela Commission on Women's Health and Reproductive Rights' is its health services arm. Apart from the health commission, there are seven other Gabriela commissions, which focus on violence against women, human rights, children and family, Filipina migrants, indigenous Filipinas, women's economic development, and international relations.

The coalition was founded on strong political ideals and aims to influence policy at the highest level. It was named after a woman leader who fought against the Spanish colonizers in the 1800s, and its leaders describe the Gabriela movement as one which "seeks to transform women into an organized political force and sees its goals as integral to the struggle for national liberation." However, Gabriela is 'grassroots' in nature. It comprises low-income and marginalized women who are primarily interested in the services and training opportunities offered by Gabriela.

Gabriela's Commission on Women's Health and Reproductive Rights was set up in 1988 by women's health professionals and women's advocates. Its primary aims are to change national thinking on women's health, encourage recognition of reproductive rights, and develop women's full and equal participation in family, community, and society. The Gabriela health commission considers the services which are currently available to women in the Philippines, including the maternity services, to be out-of-touch with the reality of women's lives. The objective is to build an alternative vision which would meet the health care needs of the majority.

Community action

A major component within Gabriela's programme of activities is work in the poor communities. Gabriela's strategy is not only to help women in poor communities to improve their own health, but also to offer education and training so that women can begin building their own clinical and community services. To date, Gabriela is running five pilot projects – three in rural communities and two in Metro Manila (Letre and Apelo).

APELO CRUZ, SQUATTER CITY

In Apelo, a squatter community in Pasay City, one of the cities that make up Metropolitan Manila, the community health workers report that only about 5% of the women have been to high school and 70% have had 5 years only of elementary education. In recent years, with falling living standards, schooling is becoming even harder to obtain.

The women of the squatter community are caught in an unending cycle of pregnancy, childbirth, and breastfeeding. Mothers of recently weaned babies may not even menstruate before discovering that they are pregnant with the next child. On top of the physical strains of child-bearing and rearing, there are the environmental risks involved in living in Apelo. It is not a healthy place. Housing consists of small, gloomy, wooden shacks crammed onto the side of a hill next to a filthy river.

Tuberculosis, coughs, colds, fever, and diarrhoea are transmitted easily in the overcrowded community. Many families in Apelo make their living from scavenging – rummaging through stinking piles of rubbish to collect either tin cans, wood, or paper. This work has its own health hazards – risk of respiratory infections, diarrhoeal disease, and tetanus. Some take drugs as a means of escaping from reality, and addiction is often associated with accidents and violence.

In theory, government health services are available to those living in Apelo because most of the country's major hospitals are located in Manila. However, transport difficulties often deter women from using the services. The journey from Apelo to the centre of Manila is time-consuming, and it is necessary to change buses at least twice. There is also the question of cost. Although doctors do not charge for their services, and contraceptives are free, patients must pay for drugs and other supplies. Completely free services are available only to those classified 'indigent' by a government social worker. Few people, even among those living in poverty in Apelo, are eligible.

Women in Apelo are well-aware that they have health problems, and they recognize the serious risk of repeated pregnancy and childbirth. They would like to be able to use good quality services, but they have serious reservations about the services currently available to them. Their views are similar to those expressed by poor women in studies conducted in Ecuador, Pakistan, Guinea-Bissau, and Bolivia (Pino *et al.*, 1990; Kazmi, 1991; Oosterbaan and Barreto da Costa, 1990; CIAES, 1991, respectively).

Women's dislike of health 'services'

Poor women and those from different ethnic groups can face poor treatment from health workers. Toyang, a community health worker, described some of the common experiences women have at the hospital. First, she says, local women felt shy and frightened by hospitals and doctors. Everyone had heard a story about being shouted at by doctors or nurses at the hospital. There was also the fear of appearing ignorant. Many women in Apelo found it difficult to read the signs in the hospital grounds, so often had problems finding their way to the right department.

Women also complained about the long periods of waiting at the hospital. They described how they would go to one department, perhaps to have their child immunized, and then find themselves referred to another department if they wanted to ask about the child's eczema, for example. The women said that they lost a great deal of time waiting to be seen. Toyang was concerned that women would sit in waiting

Victoria

Victoria is a pretty, healthy looking 25-year-old who has been living in Apelo, a squatter community of Manila Metro, for several years. She appears to be about 6 months' pregnant, but says that she will not be delivering the baby in hospital. Despite the fact that she is friendly, well-dressed, and spotlessly clean, she anticipates that she might be treated contemptuously by medical staff. She fears that she might receive the same sort of hostile treatment that her friends in Apelo have told her they received during visits to the hospital. Victoria says that she has not been for any antenatal care during this pregnancy and has not used the hospital services for any of her previous four confinements. She says that she manages things by herself without knowing her dates and without doing any tests. What she does know is that she has not menstruated since Apple, her 13-month-old baby daughter, was born.

areas worrying about whether their children at home were being taken care of, and about how many hours they were going to waste on the bus rides home. Every hour wasted at the hospital represented time lost during which the women could have been earning money.

Many women in Apelo feel that hospital staff look down on them because they are poor and uneducated. Women said that hospital staff had shouted at them. Worst of all, some women were on the receiving end of sarcastic comments about their sex lives. A typical comment of this type was: "It isn't as much fun now as when you were making the baby, is it?" Some women were chided about their inability to save enough money to cover delivery costs. This was particularly unjust as their earning capacity makes it almost impossible to save the necessary amount. Another feature of their treatment that the women complained of was that nothing was explained to them. Hospital procedures and diagnoses were bewildering, yet no explanation was provided. When the women dared to ask questions, they were given unsatisfactory answers or were scolded for being "too demanding."

These factors deter women from travelling into town for health services. There is a local government primary care unit, but women say they cannot rely on it being open, and the presence of the doctor is even less certain.

Getting organized

Community organizing in Apelo began almost as soon as the Commission itself. First, Gabriela organized discussion groups in which women started talking about their health problems and working out ways to solve them. One of the first things the women in Apelo decided was that it would be useful if one woman accompanied another on hospital visits. With someone to support them, women might find the experience less intimidating. An arrangement was therefore devised in which the more educated women volunteered to accompany other women to the hospital.

The women also decided that they needed a maternity saving scheme if they were going to deliver at the hospital. In order to help save for hospital delivery expenses, the women paid a minimum of five pesos (US 20 cents) each month into a community insurance scheme. Gabriela matched the contribution of the women peso for peso.

As a result, the women could draw out 400 pesos just before the birth of each child. Hospital expenses for a delivery totalled approximately 300 pesos, leaving 100 pesos for transport, child care, and other incidental expenses that might arise.

In order to manage these programmes, the Apelo Women's Health Association (AWHA) was formed in 1991. Currently, AWHA has a membership of 70 women, is responsible for the companion service, a community clinic, and a credit co-operative scheme, although the maternity savings scheme has been discontinued (see later). It has also started to work with a group of adolescents and with the husbands of the active association members, involving them in issues of women's health and reproductive rights.

The community clinic

The community clinic was set up in response to a request by women for local health services. Gabriela ran a 4-month community health training programme, known as the 'Basic health skills training', which several AWHA members attended. Gabriela's training programme is rigorous. Prospective health workers must give 2 days a week for 6 months to undertake the course. Besides primary health care, women learn more about their own bodies (reproductive anatomy and physiology), as well as fertility management. They also have classes on the health situation of Philippine women and how to organize women around health issues. Transportation to the training site is free, as is food and child care. The programme participants must pass written tests and a practical exam before they become health workers.

Those health workers who do pass the basic training course are given a small honorarium once they have begun to function as community health workers. The decision to pay the women health workers was taken because Gabriela believes that women's work in the health field has been consistently undervalued.

Three AWHA members have so far undertaken the training, passed the exam, and become health workers for their community. AWHA eventually found accommodation for a clinic in a windowless room in the heart of Apelo, and despite the fact that the clinic is often without electricity, it opens every day for a few hours, receiving between two and ten patients during each session.

The community health workers can diagnose and treat the most common complaints, namely coughs, colds, and diarrhoea. They prescribe simple home remedies, such as steam inhalations, cold and warm compresses, water therapy for the early stages of urinary tract infections, oral rehydration therapy (ORT), salt-water gargles for sore throats, and the use of water as an expectorant. Herbal preparations are also available from a herb garden managed jointly by Apelo and Gabriela's other community health association in Letre. The clinic pharmacy contains a supply of 'essential drugs' – generic formulations suitable for most of the needs that cannot be solved with either water or herbal treatments. Community health workers also provide information about immunization, family planning, and prenatal care. However, apart from dispensing condoms, they refer patients for actual services and in cases that they feel are serious.

Gabriela's main clinic in Metro Manila provides a broad range of services, not only for referrals from the pilot community projects, but also to Gabriela staff and members, and non-Gabriela women's groups. Services include antenatal and postpartum care, fertility management, identification and management of simple reproductive tract infections, identification and referral of other gynaecological problems, and simple drug and massage therapies. The clinic has also begun to offer birthing services for unproblematic pregnancies.

In response to a need for greater financial self-sufficiency, AWHA has set up its own credit co-operative scheme. With higher incomes, women are more likely to be able to pay for services. The credit scheme allows women to borrow 3000–5000 pesos (US$125–210) at an interest rate of 10% (half the rate they would have to pay a usurer), with an average repayment period of 6 months. The scheme started in 1994 and, to date, 32 women have borrowed a total of 92,000 pesos (US$3850), with a 76% repayment rate. The scheme is not profit-making, but Gabriela hopes that it is a first step towards AWHA autonomy. Health workers are developing book-keeping and accountancy skills, which may eventually lead them to direct access to funding partners.

AN ALTERNATIVE VISION
With this practical experience of helping to create women-determined and community-based services, Gabriela is in a strong position to begin to describe an alternative vision of a women's health programme – services that would suit the needs of the majority of women in the Philippines better than those currently available.

Gabriela's guiding principle is that women themselves must be involved in defining their health needs and the services that they would like to see provided. Specifically, Gabriela has found that if women's health status is to improve, services need to be competent, affordable, 'gender sensitive', holistic, and empowering.

Competent carers
Gabriela trains community health workers on how to deal with common problems with the help of essential drugs, herbals, and water treatments, and on cases that need to be referred. Health workers also learn about community organizing, with a view to identifying and taking action on some of the major health problems. However, Gabriela no longer considers it adequate to expend all its efforts on community health organizing while disregarding specialist referral services, and recommends that all women seek prenatal care and institutional delivery.

In order to develop skills and a perspective for competence in specialist institutions, Gabriela is currently supporting a doctor in advanced training at the Department of Obstetrics and Gynaecology at the Philippines General Hospital. The initiative represents not only a recognition of the need to provide Gabriela's health team with the highest level of technical skills, but also of the need to determine the balance between the demand for technology and medical intervention in childbirth and the resource requirements of maternal services at other levels.

Gabriela's training at all levels is guided by a new and different standard of competence. It is a standard that stresses not only medical skill, but also knowledge about the gender and class dimensions that affect women's health and lives. The aspiration is that such knowledge will result in different attitudes and behaviour towards the women who seek the services.

Affordable services

Poverty is the biggest obstacle to health for women in the Philippines. The quest for health is intimately tied up with the struggle to end overwhelming economic hardship. To achieve good health will take more than the provision of health services. Gabriela, therefore, helps women to set up co-operatives and to plan strategies against violence, crime, and drugs.

In order to make health services more affordable, Gabriela has helped support the community clinics in Apelo and Letre; some doctors in the Gabriela referral network waive their fees.

In an attempt to help women to deliver in hospital, Gabriela supported AWHA's maternity insurance scheme. However, this proved very expensive, and was benefitting richer women more than poorer community members, so it was discontinued. Instead, the community co-operative credit facility provides women with an opportunity to increase their income-creating activities.

Gender sensitivity

Gabriela is convinced of the importance of the women's perspective when defining women's health care needs and building better services. The women's perspective is built on 'gender sensitivity'. Gender refers to women's role and position in daily life, and to expectations attached to their perceived status. For example, because women are expected to be the carers, particularly of children, they become the major consumers of health services. They find themselves visiting health services not only for their own needs, but to accompany other members of the family. They have to do this as well as their daily work. The importance of the proximity of the service and hours of opening are therefore crucial issues of gender sensitivity. Another gender-sensitive issue is the attitude of medical staff towards women. As women are assumed to be of low social status, medical staff can be patronizing and expect women to wait for long periods before being seen.

Research also reveals that services relating to some of the priority health concerns identified by women, such as treatment for reproductive tract infections, infertility, complications of ageing and the menopause, and occupational and environmental health risks, are often not available to them. Gabriela believes that gender sensitivity means addressing the health problems which women themselves have identified as important.

Women at Gabriela clinics are given information about family planning and encouraged to decide for themselves as to whether or not to use fertility regulation, and which method to use. The staff are sensitive to the issue of coercion and are opposed strongly to any form of 'motivational counselling' or counting of 'acceptors'.

Holistic approach

The holistic approach is based on the idea that the body, mind, emotions, and spirit form an integrated whole, and that health is strongly related to the situation in which the individual finds herself or himself (Boston Women's Health Book Collective, 1989). The Western or 'medical' model tends not to embrace this wider vision of health. Under pressure of time, doctors tend to treat only the particular problem, disease, or injury that is presented, and may fail to respond to an underlying problem resulting from stress or living conditions.

At the Gabriela clinic, staff are well-informed about the poor conditions in which many of their patients live. Women are welcomed and given the opportunity to talk about problems other than those for which they came for treatment. A complete range of services is available at the clinic. This contrasts strongly with the maternal and child health services model, which is relevant to a woman's health needs only when she is pregnant. Reproductive health services, which represent the more holistic alternative, are relevant to a large number of women, even those outside the reproductive age group (Estrada-Claudio and Hardon, 1991). Services include, for example, treatments for menopause, stress, and infertility, as well as 'maternal' prenatal check-ups.

The holistic approach also emphasizes a sense of self-healing and community healing. Gabriela encourages women to support each other during pregnancy and delivery, and to share information among themselves about the health issues that are important to them. Ideas from traditional health-care models can then be shared. For example, some communities are rediscovering the value of herbal treatments and giving greater emphasis to the more positive aspects of the services of the TBAs, such as their willingness to allow mothers to give birth in the standing or squatting position.

Last, but not least, Gabriela's holistic approach recognizes the significance of poverty and injustice as causes of ill-health. In response, it provides both training for community organizing and information on political and economic aspects of life in the Philippines. Gabriela's regular radio broadcasts, for example, cover not only the various aspects of reproductive health, but also feature tax and price changes that create special burdens for poor communities.

Empowerment

Health can only be achieved if people feel capable and responsible for their own lives. Unfortunately, contact with some medical institutions can have the opposite effect on both women and men. As patients, part of women's fear and powerlessness is caused by lack of knowledge and lack of opportunity to take part in the decisions being taken on their behalf. When asked, women typically say that they would prefer to spend labour active and on their feet, in a warm and caring environment, with loved ones around them. Medical institutions seldom allow this. Medical professionals often consider the patient's subjective experience to be much less important than a doctor's clinical experience.

Gabriela's staff are concerned to show their patients respect and to instil in them a sense that their time, their feelings, and their experiences are important. Staff try to explain delays to women who have to wait, and aim to ensure that all health problems can be dealt with at the same place and at the same time. During an appointment for immunization for her child, for example, a woman can also discuss her feelings of stress, or receive family planning information or services.

Another attempt to empower women comes through Gabriela's training programmes. Community organizers structure the training modules on reproductive health to gradually build up women's knowledge of their own physiology. Without this basic knowledge, attempts to inform women about the different modes of action of fertility regulation would be impossible. The programmes often have an empowering effect. According to one member of staff (Berer, 1993):

> *What is interesting is that very often it is not what we teach that has helped women, but the mere fact that we have considered them worthwhile teaching or organizing .... I have seen women actually cry during our assessments, not because of the gains achieved, but merely because someone encouraged them to take political action and accorded them equal value with men.*

Another important component in efforts to empower women is through building community action. Gabriela's health commission works closely with other commissions to share valuable experiences in community initiatives. Gabriela also works closely with Samakana, an organization of urban poor housewives and working women which has set up a number of community co-operatives. Samakana has produced training programmes and booklets on women's and national issues. These resources are used by women involved in Gabriela's health programmes.

CAMPAIGNING AND ALLIANCE BUILDING

One of the long-term aims of Gabriela is to bring about changes in national thinking on women's health and reproductive rights. Gabriela therefore encourages all women to demand the convenient, affordable, dignified, and supportive health services that they want.

Over 150 people from Apelo took part in the International Day of Action for Women's Health on 28th May 1994. The AWHA used it as an opportunity to launch its drama presentation on the pressing issues for women in the localities. On Women's Day (8th March) in 1994, women from Apelo and the other pilot urban community in Letre helped members of Gabriela's health staff to provide first aid services for other participants.

Gabriela has been organizing this type of event ever since the launch of the International Day of Action for Women's Health in 1988. It is a member of the Women's Global Network for Reproductive Rights (WGNRR), the group which launched the initiative. In May 1992 Gabriela organized a month-long nation-wide campaign on pregnancy-related mortality. The Gabriela health commission has recommended to the government that May 28th should be declared a National Day of Action for Women's Health.

Gabriela attempts to raise the issues by working closely with other active groups. The Gabriela health commission was part of a seven-group alliance organizing committee for the 'Sixth International Women and Health Meeting' in November 1990. It is also part of an alliance of about 20 local organizations involved in health and reproductive rights, as well as a national AIDS–NGO (non-governmental organization) network.

PROBLEMS AND CHALLENGES

The services of Gabriela's health commission make only a very small contribution to the totality of services required by women in the Philippines. The community clinics in Apelo and Letre are estimated to take just over 1000 patient per year each, and the Gabriela clinic in Metro Manila receives approximately 1200 patient visits.

Despite the input by Gabriela within the Apelo community since 1988, the membership of AWHA is only 70 women out of a total community of several thousand. Gabriela staff believe that the patronizing treatment to which women are generally subjected creates a passivity that makes it difficult to involve them in community organizing. Gabriela is fully aware that it has not discovered the key to creating mass mobilization of poor women for health action.

While management skills and responsibilities for the clinic and the credit co-operative are slowly being transferred to the health workers and AWHA, there is no clear strategy on which to plan a pull-out from Apelo. Gabriela continues to provide a 50% subsidy on the drugs supplied to the clinic, and subsidizes the costs of women who need to be referred to other health facilities. This financial burden is added to insecurity with regard to the funding of the Gabriela clinic, which has never been assured a long-term commitment.

As well as the limits of Gabriela staff time, there is the continuing need for upgrading the capacity and competence of staff. The doctors, midwives, and nurses who run the programmes have often come from either economically disadvantaged or activist backgrounds, or both, and have therefore had to devote less time and effort to the improvement of their professional skills.

There are also political challenges. Gabriela is faced with a national situation which is fraught with difficulties. Often, it seems that any attention given by the government to family planning is effectively nullified by the Roman Catholic Church. Reproductive rights that exist need to be vigilantly defended. As new conservative initiatives arise, campaign responses are needed.

Next year, there are plans to evaluate the entire Gabriela health programme. Despite years of experience and the growing framework and guidelines for a more woman-centred programme, indicators for programme assessment have not yet been identified.

ACHIEVEMENTS

Gabriela's greatest achievement has been in its creation of an alternative vision of women's health services. It is a vision of a health service that would meet the needs of the majority. Based on the concept of reproductive rights, it would ensure that women had the right to self-determination with regard to their own bodies. It would ensure much greater involvement of women in planning and decision-making.

In developing this vision of a quality service for all, Gabriela has shown that the experience of female gender produces a women's perspective. Problems and needs identified in the Apelo community echoed with those of researchers as far away as Bolivia, Guinea Bissau, and Pakistan.

If it were needed, this identification of the women's perspective confirms the necessity for women to play a greater part in developing the on-going priorities of health services. If women are to participate fully and equally, more women need to be trained and appointed to senior positions.

Gabriela has also been able to promote its alternative vision. Campaign work, both nationally and internationally, has drawn attention to maternal mortality and morbidity, and to abortion as a public health issue. This advocacy for women's health has created an awareness of the need for alternative visions. As more governments and groups recognize that need, Gabriela will be able to provide guidance on women's health services of the future.

REFERENCES

Berer, M. (1993) *Women's Groups, NGOs and Safe Motherhood*. Maternal Health and Safe Motherhood Programme, Division of Family Health, World Health Organization, Geneva.

Bongga, D.C. (1992) *State of the National Health: Adequacy of Nutrition*. Paper presented at the 'Roundtable Discussion on the National Health and Health Services' sponsored by the Institute of Human Rights, UP Law Center, Manila.

Boston Women's Health Book Collective (1989) *The New Our Bodies, Ourselves*. British edition by Phillips, A. and Rakusen, J. The Penguin Group, London.

CIAES (1991) *Qualitative Research on Knowledge, Attitudes, and Practices Related to Women's Reproductive Health*. Working Paper No. 9, MotherCare Project, Center for Health Research, Consultation and Education, Cochabamba, Bolivia.

Department of Health (1989) *Health Intelligence Service*. Philippine Health Statistics, Manila.

Dixon-Mueller, R. and Germain, A. (1994) Population policy and feminist political action in three developing countries. In: Finkle, J.L. and McIntosh, C.A. (eds), *The New Politics of Population*, a supplement to *Population and Development Review*, Volume 20. The Population Council, New York.

Estrada-Claudio, S. (1992) *Country Report for the Philippines*. A paper prepared for the Asian Regional Meeting on Women's Perspectives on the Selection and Introduction of Fertility-Regulating Technologies, sponsored by the World Health Organization, Manila.

Estrada-Claudio, S. and Hardon, A. (1991) User-perspectives on fertility regulation technologies and services: A research framework. *Health Alert*, **122**: 265–272.

Kazmi, S. (1991) *Safe Motherhood: Consumer Viewpoints, Sample Survey*. Marketing and Research Consultant (MARC), Association of Business and Professional and Agricultural Women, Pakistan. Unpublished.

Miralao, V.A. and Engracia, L.T. (1989) In the throes of transition: Fertility trends and patterns in the Philippines. *Philippine Sociological Review*, **37**(3–4).

Oosterbaan, M. and Barreto da Costa, M.V. (1990) *Motherhood in Guinea-Bissau: What Women Know about the Risks: An Anthropological Study*. Available in MSM database, Maternal Health and Safe Motherhood programme, World Health Organization, Geneva.

Pino, M.A. *et al.* (1990) *Alternative Approaches to Improve the Coverage and Quality of Maternal Health Care in Ecuador*. Available in MSM database, Maternal Health and Safe Motherhood programme, World Health Organization, Geneva.

Raymundo, C.M. (1987) *Risks of Motherhood among the Urban Poor*. Paper presented to the National Conference on Safe Motherhood, Manila.

SMS (1993) *Philippines National Safe Motherhood Survey 1993*. National Statistics Office, Manila, Philippines, and Macro International, Calverton, USA.

Tan, M.L. (1989) *Health Alert*, **95**: 20

Tan, M.L. (1992) Women's health in the Philippines, a critical analysis. *Health Alert*, **VIII**: 129–130.

UNICEF (1991) *State of the World's Children, 1991*. Oxford University Press, Oxford.

UNICEF (1994) *State of the World's Children, 1994*. Oxford University Press, Oxford.

CHAPTER 12

Woman-Led Midwifery: The Development of a New Midwifery Philosophy in Britain

Nicky Leap

INTRODUCTION

The concept of 'woman-led maternity care' has been endorsed by various British Government reports in recent years (House of Commons Health Committee, 1992; Department of Health, 1992, 1993) and it has been recognized that midwifery should be driven by a philosophy that enables child-bearing women to have "choice, control and continuity of care" (Hutton, 1994). This represents a move away from the somewhat rigid authoritarianism associated with the drive to professionalize midwifery. It has come about in a political climate influenced by feminism, by consumerism, and, in recent years, by a shift away from the values of collective responsibility, as enshrined in the National Health Service (NHS), towards a neo-liberalist ideology that places the rights of the individual uppermost within a market economy.

In this chapter the development of the concept of 'woman-led care' is traced and how one group of midwives in an inner-city area of south-east London translated this into practice is examined.

THE PROFESSIONALIZATION OF MIDWIFERY IN BRITAIN

In Britain until the early decades of the twentieth century, the majority of women were attended in childbirth by a local woman, whom they knew well. She was the person called upon when a woman was in labour or if a dead body needed to be laid out (Leap and Hunter, 1993):

> *She saw you into the world and she saw you out the other end .... It was just the thing that you called for her.*

This woman was known by local people as 'the midwife', although official documentation in the first half of this century refers to her as 'the handywoman', possibly because many midwives were elderly widows who also gained a small living from taking on domestic tasks, such as tending the sick, taking in washing, and child care.

The struggle to professionalize midwifery in Britain has been well-documented (Donnison, 1977; Towler and Bramall, 1986). In the early part of this century, the new trained, professional midwife was at pains to be seen as a respectable member of the medical professions. She therefore liked to be referred to as 'the nurse', not wanting to be associated with the person referred to as 'the midwife', who tended to be illiterate and working class (Leap and Hunter, 1993). As part of the campaign to build a respectable profession for middle- and upper-class women, the untrained midwives were often scorned and derided; they were denied the opportunity to train and, eventually, they were hounded out of midwifery by restrictive and punitive legislation (Heagerty, 1990).

Early midwifery legislation was negotiated with the understanding that midwives would refer all cases that were not strictly 'normal' to doctors, thereby ensuring a steady income for doctors and minimizing any professional threat to the medical profession. Strict supervisory mechanisms were employed to enforce legislation, and midwives were expected to learn and practise according to inflexible rules designed by the medical profession.

There is some evidence that midwives saw it as their crusade to instruct 'the foolish poor' and to inculcate working-class people with middle-class values. An authoritarian approach was rewarded and seen as being appropriate behaviour, and the idea of keeping a professional distance was encouraged (Leap and Hunter, 1993). As late as 1985, midwives were being encouraged in a leading textbook to (Myles, 1985):

> Counteract liberal attitudes to sexuality [and the] threatened breakdown of the family, [and to] counsel [parents about] moral codes and high ideals since they are at fault through ignorance.

By the early 1980s, the number of women giving birth at home had fallen to 1% and many midwives could see their role being reduced to that of an obstetric nurse whose job was to assist doctors with 'managing' a childbirth dominated by technology and a mechanized approach. However, in such a climate, support and campaign groups, such as the Association for Improvements in Maternity Services (AIMS), the National Childbirth Trust (NCT), the Active Birth Movement, and the Society to Support Home Confinements, gathered popular support from women who were not prepared to tolerate a system that left many feeling powerless.

THE VISION: PROPOSALS FOR THE FUTURE OF THE MATERNITY SERVICES FROM THE ASSOCIATION OF RADICAL MIDWIVES

In 1986 the Association of Radical Midwives (ARM) proposed a 'vision' for the maternity services of the future (ARM, 1986). They were motivated by a concern to change a system that seemed predisposed towards fragmented, medicalized, impersonal care: a system that under-utilized midwives' skills and prevented midwives from feeling that they were "practitioners in their own right."

The basic principles from which the proposals in *The Vision* evolved were:

- The relationship between mother and midwife is fundamental to good midwifery care
- The mother is the central person in the process of care.

- Informed choice in childbirth for women.
- Full utilization of midwives' skills.
- Continuity of care for all child-bearing women.
- Community-based care.
- Accountability of services to those receiving them.
- Care should do no harm to mother and baby.

The Vision proposed a system that would allow the majority of midwives to work in community-based group practices, taking on the total care for most of the 85% of women who do not have complicated pregnancies. It was suggested that 30–40% of midwives would be in hospital-based teams, working alongside consultant obstetricians providing care for those women who needed hospital attention. Flexible working arrangements, including job sharing, were recommended, as were antenatal and postnatal support groups. Emphasis was placed on the idea that midwives should be the first point of entry into care for all pregnant women, thus enabling a full choice of options to be offered. To promote this, midwives should be visible in their communities, they should offer pregnancy testing, and their services should be publicized widely.

THE HOUSE OF COMMONS HEALTH COMMITTEE *SECOND REPORT – MATERNITY SERVICES*

Although *The Vision* was a booklet published by a small organization, subsequent documents from both statutory and professional bodies can be seen to have incorporated both its ideology and many of its practical suggestions. Indeed, strong echoes of *The Vision* are apparent in the House of Commons Health Committee's *Second Report – Maternity Services* (House of Commons Health Committee, 1992). The Health Committee's Report was greeted with enthusiasm by childbirth organizations and midwives, since its overall message was that maternity services should be fashioned around the needs of women and their families, that a medical model of care was inappropriate in such circumstances, and that there should be recognition of the midwife's skills.

CHANGING CHILDBIRTH

The government's main response to the Health Committee's Report on maternity services was to set up a task force to review maternity services and make recommendations for the future. While *Changing Childbirth* (Department of Health, 1993) was less radical in its proposals than its predecessor, it acknowledged the themes of "choice, control, and continuity of care" and recommended a service that was "kinder, more welcoming and more supportive to the women whose needs it is designed to meet." Ten key indicators were identified which would demonstrate that the report's recommendations had been put into place within 5 years:

1. All women should be entitled to carry their own notes.
2. Every woman should know one midwife who ensures continuity of her midwifery care – the 'named midwife'.
3. At least 30% of women should have the midwife as the lead professional.
4. Every woman should know the lead professional who has a key role in the

planning and provision of her care.

5. At least 75% of women should know the person who cares for them during their delivery.
6. Midwives should have direct access to some beds in all maternity units.
7. At least 30% of women delivered in a maternity unit should be admitted under management of the midwife.
8. The total number of antenatal visits for women with uncomplicated pregnancies should have been reviewed in the light of the available evidence and the guidelines of the Royal College of Obstetricians & Gynaecologists (RCOG, 1982).
9. All front-line ambulances should have a paramedic able to support a midwife who needs to transfer a woman to hospital in an emergency.
10. All women should have access to information about the services available in their locality.

THE SOUTH-EAST LONDON MIDWIFERY GROUP PRACTICE (SELMGP)

It was in this climate of innovation, beginning with *The Vision* and leading to *Changing Childbirth*, that a midwifery group practice evolved in south-east London. SELMGP was first set up by independent ('independent' refers to the fact that the midwives were self-employed, not employed by an NHS Trust or hospital) midwives who were working in the same geographical area and were drawn together both by the practical need to provide support and midwifery cover for each other and by a common philosophy (see the following boxes).

Philosophy of SELMGP

SELMGP defined its philosophy as:

- Midwifery care is a trusting partnership of equals between the woman and her carers.
- Pregnancy and childbirth are seen as a normal part of a woman's life within her social context.
- Each woman is entitled to get to know the midwives caring for her throughout her pregnancy and childbirth, regardless of recognized 'risk factors', complications, or place of birth.
- Women should be enabled to give birth to healthy babies in a normal, safe, and satisfying way in the place of their choice.
- Each pregnant woman books with two midwives who undertake all her midwifery care.
- The midwife 'follows the woman', thereby enabling care either at home or in hospital, appropriate to the woman's needs and choices.
- SELMGP believes in the principles of the NHS and feel that all women should have access to this type of care, free at the point of service, regardless of whether or not they can afford to pay.

Objectives of SELMGP

FOR THE WOMEN

- To ensure, as far as possible, the birth of a mature, live, healthy infant.
- To prepare the woman for labour, birth, and the care and feeding of her child.
- To provide women and their partners with information about the choices concerning the care given during pregnancy, labour, and the postnatal period.
- To enable the woman and her partner to be responsible equally with the midwife and the medical practitioners for her physical health and emotional well-being before, during, and after pregnancy.
- To provide continuity of care for women, with two named midwives who will remain responsible for the midwifery care throughout pregnancy, labour, and the postnatal period (up to 28 days).
- To detect conditions which may endanger or affect the future health of the mother or baby and to refer the woman to the appropriate practitioner.
- To ensure that the birth of the baby is as emotionally satisfying as possible for the mother, and also a rewarding experience for the whole family.
- To encourage women to evaluate the care given during pregnancy, labour, and the postnatal period, and to make changes accordingly.

FOR THE MIDWIVES

- To enable midwives to take full responsibility for the midwifery care of the named women.
- To enable midwives to listen to and respect the needs of women.
- To enable midwives to be accountable to the women in their care.
- To foster mutual trust and respect between midwives and the women in their care.
- To foster mutual trust and respect between midwives and other practitioners.
- To enable midwives to design their own working practice.
- To enable midwives to choose the size of the case-load.
- To enable midwives to manage their own time as appropriate to individual commitments.
- To enhance job satisfaction.
- To improve the retention of midwives in midwifery practice.
- To maintain and develop a wide range of clinical midwifery skills.
- To provide a supportive learning environment for student midwives and other practitioners.

One of the intentions of SELMGP was to see if the excellent outcomes associated with the independent midwifery care of a predominantly middle-class population (Weig, 1993) could be maintained when the case-load addressed the issues of inner-city deprivation and inequalities in health. The statistics were encouraging. Of 506 births, 45% of which were women having their first babies and over 25% of which were women over the age of 35, the following emerged:

- Of the 506 women, 69 planned to have their babies in hospital; of these 13 decided during labour to have their babies at home as things were obviously going well.

- Of the 437 women who planned to give birth at home, 69 (16%) ended up giving birth in hospital.
- The total home birth rate was 75%.
- The overall rate of spontaneous vaginal births was 87.8%. The caesarean section rate was 6.7%, forceps and ventouse rate was 5.5%.
- Augmentation of labour was needed by 37 women (7.3%).
- The episiotomy rate for births at home was 1%. In hospital, the rate was 7%, including all instrumental births.
- No perineal tears occurred in 40% of the women and 39% had tears that did not need suturing; thus, the total rate for women who did not require perineal suturing was 79%.
- No pharmacological analgesia was used by 74% of the women during labour (epidural rate, 11%; pethidine, 1%; Entonox, 11%; combination of these, 3%).
- The breastfeeding rate at discharge, 28 days after the birth, was 96.4%.

These statistics were similar to data on over 1000 births provided by the birth registers of independent midwives (Weig, 1993).

MIDWIFERY GROUP PRACTICE WITH A HEALTH AUTHORITY CONTRACT

In April 1994, SELMGP became the first midwifery group practice to obtain a contract with a local health authority with National Health Service (NHS) funding. The plan was for each full-time midwife to have a case-load of 35 women for whom she was to be the primary midwife. She would also be involved in the care of another 35 women as secondary or back-up midwife. The midwives decided to arrange their work so that, rather than having 2 days off a week, they would be on call for agreed months of the year with extended blocks of holiday totalling 3 months. The usual pattern would be 3 months on-call and 1 month off. Thus, an individual midwife's case-load would consist of women whose babies were due in the time when she could guarantee to be on call. Working with a case-load means that midwifery care 'follows the woman', and midwives arrange their own working hours to accommodate this rather than following a traditional 'shift work' arrangement.

The eight midwives began practising, in partnership with a practice manager, from premises based in a busy community centre in Deptford, an inner-city area of south-east London. A walk-in shop-front opens on to a pedestrian precinct where, three times a week, there is a busy market. Local groups meet and socialize at the community centre, particularly in the cafe which is run as a training centre for people with learning difficulties. Other projects in the building include a children and parents centre, a crèche, a welfare rights project, and various women's projects, all of which offer the midwives the opportunity for good liaison with other workers in the local community.

SELMGP offers free pregnancy testing, antenatal and postnatal groups, walk-in advice and information, referral for pregnancy counselling, a library service, and continuity of midwifery care that is free at the point of service. The practice undertakes the total midwifery care of approximately 200 women per year. Each woman is allocated two midwives who look after her throughout her pregnancy, labour, and the first month of her baby's life, thus enabling a trusting relationship to develop. Women who are most vulnerable in terms of socio-economic need are targeted by the project.

The midwives work with women who are booked for either hospital or home birth. Women are encouraged to make final decisions about the place of birth when they are in labour. If all is going well, many women decide to stay at home; if labour is not straightforward or the woman wants to go to hospital, the midwives stay with her in hospital throughout her labour and the first few hours after birth. The home birth rate for the SELMGP is high, with consistently good outcomes and appropriate use of hospitals for transfer.

The SELMGP case-load includes women with known medical and obstetric complications, as these women are often the most in need of continuity of midwifery care and support. The midwives in the group practice have developed excellent liaison with other health professionals, are able to make direct referrals to other practitioners, and have direct use of laboratory and ultrasound facilities at local hospitals.

The midwives in the SELMGP are used to working together as autonomous practitioners responsible for their own practice, business administration, and finances. They meet regularly for support, peer review, skill-sharing, and to discuss organizational matters. The SELMGP has an advisory group composed of 50% users of the service and 50% professionals with relevant expertise. This group undertakes to monitor the work of the practice, including complaints.

Client-led antenatal and postnatal groups

Free weekly antenatal and postnatal groups are run as described in a video made by women in the groups (Leap, 1992a). These include women-only groups and groups that include partners. Women can come to the antenatal groups at any stage of their pregnancy; in any one group there will be a mixture of women in early and late pregnancy, women having first and subsequent babies, and women with a wide range of age and experience. The groups provide an opportunity for women to direct their own learning, and to find out about the things that are relevant and pertinent to their lives. There is no set agenda and the midwife acts as a group facilitator who picks up on relevant topics as they emerge.

Each woman returns to the group in the early weeks after she has had her baby and tells her birth story. These stories stimulate discussion and provide a wide range of information that is based on real situations. Close friendships can develop in the antenatal group and later in the postnatal group, which can help to break down the isolation of new motherhood.

Work with the community from Vietnam

The SELMGP is building strong links with the local Vietnamese community. There are over 400 families from Vietnam living in the area, the majority of whom arrived in Britain after spending several years in refugee camps in Hong Kong. Unemployment and poverty, compounded by language difficulties, isolation, and community fragmentation make life very hard for many of these families. For those who had previous babies in Hong Kong and Vietnam, there are often tales of the worst, most brutal aspects of exported Western obstetric practice, which have left their mark. Midwifery continuity-of-care can make a vital difference to the experience of child-bearing for the women from Vietnam, many of whom are keen to have their babies at home, a choice rarely offered to them.

The SELMGP involvement with this community extends beyond the birth of the baby to taking women to register their babies, supporting women through miscarriage and termination of pregnancy, and developing links with the local interpreting service. Close liaison with a local support group for women from Vietnam has led to the setting up of a maternity link project, which will enable health advocates to work alongside the midwives.

SELMGP as a resource

SELMGP provides a national and international resource for those interested in this type of midwifery practice through:

- Lecturing at national and international conferences, study days, and midwifery colleges.
- Organizing a national forum, based at the Royal College of Midwives, for those involved in implementing midwifery case-load practice.
- Liaising with universities to design and implement learning packages used to update qualified midwives.
- Acting as consultants for local hospitals when they set up midwifery group practices.
- Being advisors to the National Health Service Management Executive.
- Running monthly workshops for interested midwives who work throughout the UK.
- Providing placements for both midwives and students who wish to experience this type of midwifery practice.
- Hosting midwives from other countries, e.g., the United States, Australia, New Zealand, Canada, the Netherlands.
- Responding to media interest and making regular contributions to the midwifery press.
- Running courses for midwives and general practitioners on facilitating home births.

WOMAN-LED MIDWIFERY IN PRACTICE

Much has been written about 'empowerment' in recent years, and there appears to be a common understanding that an important aim of the midwife is to facilitate the empowerment of women through their experiences of pregnancy, birth, and parenting. It has also been recognized that midwives cannot facilitate the empowerment of women if they are disempowered themselves (Jamieson, 1994).

The experience of SELMGP suggests that the concept of enabling or empowering through doing as little as possible is an important component of the art of midwifery in all settings. So often midwives gain kudos from the 'doing' things, while the simple 'with-woman' skills are hard to quantify or to describe, and therefore often receive little acknowledgement. It is useful to look in chronological order at the interaction that a midwife has with a pregnant woman and her family, to identify some of the styles of practice that fit with the philosophy of woman-led midwifery.

The idea of encouraging women to share the task of filling in their booking notes is beginning to attract wider attention in Britain. In SELMGP, women are encouraged to write their own antenatal and postnatal record if they want to. The midwives are learning to write full notes that are descriptive and meaningful to the women, avoiding abbreviations, using sentences, and including the woman's name wherever possible.

During the antenatal period the SELMGP midwives are trying to move away from a task-orientated approach and develop the ability to listen to women. Some midwives are developing a style of practice which avoids routine listening to the fetal heart unless the woman specifically asks for this or there are concerns about the baby's well-being. Such midwives ask the woman how she thinks the baby is – how and when it is moving, how does she think her baby is growing. This approach encourages women to see themselves as the main source of monitoring of their baby's well-being, so reducing the dependency on professional expertise where it is not needed.

When helping women to make choices about labour, I would argue that midwives need to minimize the 'menu' approach – giving women huge lists of possibilities and options to choose from. Instead, a 'wait and see' and 'keep your options open' policy can be more useful. The important message for women is that they *will* know at the time. Similarly, women need to know that they *will* know the most appropriate way to breathe in labour, the most appropriate noises to make, the most appropriate way to move, and the positions to adopt that will help the normal process and enable them to cope with pain. Women do not need to be taught these methods of responding to labour.

Talking about pain, as opposed to 'pain relief', is an important starting point. The message can be that in uncomplicated labour where the baby is in a good position the uterus works efficiently so there will not be pain that cannot be coped with. This is far more positive than asking what type of pain relief a woman wants followed by the menu of misnamed methods of 'pain relief', and their benefits and risks.

The emphasis on 'doing' tasks not only occurs in hospitals. In some settings, the 'active management of labour' has taken place using one or other of the so-called 'complementary' therapies. If, at the end of the day, after an uncomplicated labour, a woman says, "I couldn't have done it without the [for example] homeopathy, or the acupuncture, or indeed the midwife," then at some level she has given away the power that is hers by right. The feeling that she has done something unbelievably clever, powerful, and demanding is diminished by an investment outside of herself.

Working at developing a midwifery that places the woman centre stage means that midwives must develop listening skills and the ability to take on a quietly supportive role. In hospital, a midwife who is not previously acquainted with a woman often works hard at building trust and friendship in the short time that they are thrown together. This requires a lot of 'doing' things – lots of talking, finding common ground, jokes, massage, eye contact, loving attention, sitting beside the woman throughout labour muttering encouragement with the sponge and iced water – indeed, this is generally what people think being 'with woman' is all about.

When midwives come to know a woman throughout pregnancy, however, a different approach often develops. The midwife will have met the people the woman has chosen to support her in labour – usually a partner, close friends, or family. She will make sure that *these* people are the ones who do all the eye contact, the massage, and the loving attention during labour. Midwives in this situation tend to sit in a corner of the room in watchful anticipation during labour. On the whole, they are very quiet and non-directive. They have been able to develop an approach that minimizes disturbance, intervention, direction, and authority; and maximizes the potential for physiology, common sense, and instinct to prevail. This approach places trust in the expertise of child-bearing women, which inevitably involves a shift of power towards the child-bearing woman.

In labour, the midwife can, without resorting to regular vaginal examinations, develop skills to assess how labour is progressing through watching, listening, and taking cues from the woman. Studies have shown that when audio tape or video tape recordings of labouring women are played to midwives, they are very accurate in assessing the relevant stages of labour (McKay and Roberts, 1990; Baker and Kenner, 1993). This skill applied even to those who had only been qualified a couple of years (Baker and Kenner, 1993).

The SELMGP midwives have found it very useful to arrange a meeting, at about 36 weeks of pregnancy, with the people who are likely to be at the woman's labour. They look at pictures of births together, describing the normal process of labour, covering topics such as potential roles, taking cues from the labouring woman, minimizing disturbance, and those tasks and behaviours that might be helpful, particularly in enabling women to cope with pain. This makes people confident about their role and ensures that everyone involved has a basic understanding of the process of normal labour and the vocabulary involved. It also means that people are not meeting the midwives for the first time during the woman's labour. Preparing in this way optimizes the potential for the woman to labour in a supportive environment where stimulation to the senses and disturbance are minimized, which enables the hormones of labour to work effectively, including the body's pain-modifying opiates (Odent, 1984; Robertson, 1994).

Midwives need to respect the extraordinary nature and intricacy of the many interacting hormonal cascades and surging polypeptide chains that trigger feedback mechanisms in a swirling dance of purpose. Understanding even a small part of the mechanisms involved can increase a midwife's wonder and encourage her to work hard at avoiding disturbance in the form of light, sound, touch, and smell. (Even the very presence of the midwife may disturb, at times.)

During labour, the midwife can develop her role as a 'safety net', knowing when to act, when to make suggestions, when to encourage, but, more importantly, when not to do any of these things. Midwives have to work hard against the notion that they should be directing proceedings. This means rejecting the sort of power that is associated with words like *control, manage, supervise, conduct*, and *allow*. These are used in the language of 'confinement' and removing them from our vocabulary could be a good starting point to shift power from birth attendants to women (Bastion, 1992; Leap 1992b).

For example, when a midwife is tempted to say something like, "I had a nice delivery last night," she should stop and remember that it is the woman who delivers her baby, not the midwife. It may not be too difficult to substitute the noun 'birth' for 'delivery', but sometimes the 'doing' words are harder to replace. Some midwives try to talk about 'attending' women as a substitute for 'delivering'. The alternative term 'catching' babies may be seen as trivializing the process. Perhaps a phrase that can be found in other languages, 'receiving' the baby, is more appropriate.

For a woman, a crucial part of the act of giving birth is picking up the baby. Apart from the fact that this puts her in an ideal position to deliver her placenta, it allows the woman control of the act of giving birth. Midwives know that, very often, women do not want to pick up their babies straight away. They need time to recover from a process which often feels as though it is nothing to do with babies. Women reach out tentatively, exclaiming and saying things like, "Oh, it's a baby!", "Is it mine?", "Is it all right?". It may be several minutes, or even longer, before the woman reaches down to pick up her baby, during which time the midwife can have handed over warmed towels or a heating pad and made quiet reminders, if needed, about preventing the baby from getting cold. With the ensuing counting of toes and fingers and the pouring over the minutiae of physical uniqueness and familial likeness, begins the process of the woman checking her own baby's well-being that is so important an aspect of parenting – the mother as that particular baby's expert.

In the postnatal period, routine checks can usually be avoided by asking women simple, open-ended questions and listening to the answers. For example, examining perineal wounds should arguably only happen if the woman expresses concern. In such circumstances, a check can be made together, using a mirror, so that the woman is directly involved in monitoring her healing and well-being. Once again, midwives need to trust that healthy women have bodies that will heal well. It could be argued that even suggesting routine herbal compresses undermines this message.

Similarly, midwives usually learn more from asking women questions about their baby than carrying out 'strip searches'. Again, this is about giving mothers the message that they are their baby's expert. Helping women to gain confidence as new mothers is about minimizing the information given by professionals, and waiting to be asked when it is felt needed by the woman. It is also about the midwife having networking skills that enable her to put women in touch with each other, either individually or through relevant support groups.

I suspect that, throughout history, there have always been midwives who have understood the art of doing as little as possible. Unfortunately, the recent professionalization of midwifery in Britain in the twentieth century has often led to midwives seeing themselves as authority figures, even when based in the community (Leap and Hunter, 1993). The key to creating a new, woman-centred midwifery may well lie in attempting to uphold the advice found in the *Tao Te Ching*, written over 2500 years ago (Heider, 1986):

> You are a midwife: you are assisting at someone else's birth. Do good without show or fuss. Facilitate what is happening rather than what you think ought to be happening. If you must take the lead, lead so that the mother is helped, yet still free and in charge. When the baby is born, the mother will rightly say: "We did it ourselves!"

Whatever structures we design in order to be midwives, to be 'with woman', an underlying philosophy that believes in woman-led care will produce situations in which it is possible for women to feel empowered by the experience of childbirth, situations where the mother will rightly say: "We did it ourselves!"

REFERENCES

ARM (1986) *The Vision: Proposals for the Future of the Maternity Services.* Association of Radical Midwives, Ormskirk, Lancashire.

Baker, A. and Kenner, A.N. (1993) Communication of pain: Vocalization as an indicator of the stage of labour. *Australian and New Zealand Journal of Obstetrics and Gynaecology*, **33**(4): 384–385.

Bastion, H. (1992) Confined, managed, and delivered: The language of obstetrics. *British Journal of Obstetrics and Gynaecology*, February: **99**: 92–93.

Department of Health (1992) *Maternity Services: Government Response to the Second Report from the Health Committee, Session 1991–92.* Cmnd 2018, HMSO, London.

Department of Health (1993) *Changing Childbirth.* HMSO, London.

Donnison, J. (1977) *Midwives and Medical Men.* Heinemann, London.

Heagerty, B. (1990) *Class, Gender, and Professionalization: The Struggle for British Midwifery, 1900–1936.* Unpublished dissertation. Available at the Royal College of Midwives Library (reference only), London.

Heider, J. (ed.) (1986) *The Tao of Leadership.* Wildwood House.

Hobbs, L. (1993) *The Independent Midwife: A Guide to Independent Midwifery Practice.* Books for Midwives Press, London.

House of Commons Health Committee (1992) *Second Report – Maternity Services.* HMSO, London.

Hutton, E. (1994) What women want from midwives. *British Journal of Midwifery*, **2**(12): 608–611.

Jamieson, L. (1994) Midwife empowerment through education. *British Journal of Midwifery*, **2**(2): 47–48.

Leap, N. (1992a) *Helping You to Make Your Own Decisions: Antenatal and Postnatal Groups in Deptford, SE London.* VHS Video, 25 minutes. Available from SELMGP, The Albany, Douglas Way, Deptford, London SE8 4AG.

Leap, N. (1992b) The power of words. *Nursing Times*, **88**(21): 60–61.

Leap, N. and Hunter, B. (1993) *The Midwife's Tale: An Oral History from Handywoman to Professional Midwife.* Scarlet Press, London.

McKay, S. and Roberts, J. (1990) Obstetrics by ear: Maternal and care giver perceptions of the meaning of maternal sounds during second stage labor. *Journal of Nurse Midwifery*, **35**(5): 266–273.

Myles, M. (1981) *Textbook for Midwives: With Modern Concepts of Obstetric and Neonatal Care*, 9th edn. Churchill Livingstone, London.

Odent, M. (1984) *Birth Reborn: What Birth Can and Should Be*. Souvenir Press, London.

RCOG (1982) *Report of the RCOG Working Party on Antenatal and Intrapartum Care*. Royal College of Obstetricians and Gynaecologists, London.

Robertson, A. (1994) *Empowering Women: Teaching Active Birth in the 1990s*. Ace Graphics, NSW, Australia.

Towler, J. and Bramall, L. (1986) *Midwives in History and Society*. Croom Helm, London.

Weig, M. (1993) *Audit of Independent Midwifery 1980–1991*. The Royal College of Midwives, London.

CHAPTER

13

The Quality of Care in Maternal and Reproductive Health Services: Definition, Assessment, and Improvement

Patricia Semeraro and **Barbara S. Mensch**

INTRODUCTION

> *The notion of quality of care is implicit in any medical action. Health professionals view themselves as individuals who dedicate their lives to prevent disease, improve health, and care for the ill. Every physician, nurse, and midwife wants to see him/herself and be seen by others as a good professional. To be good and to do good means to be able to provide care of good quality. (Faundes, 1990.)*

There has been a growing recognition of the need to assess the quality of health services in developing countries (Das Gupta, 1989; United Nations, 1991). The World Health Organization (WHO) has outlined approaches and developed protocols for the evaluation of primary health care services in such countries (Roemer and Montoya-Aguilar, 1988). Within the specific field of maternal health services, a Subcommittee on Quality of Care Indicators in Family Planning Service Delivery was formed several years ago to establish guidelines for measuring the quality of care in the provision of family planning services (Subcommittee on Quality Indicators in Family Planning Service Delivery, 1990). In the period since then, donors, international organizations, local NGOs, and, to a lesser extent, government health ministries have begun to devote resources to diagnosing and improving the quality of reproductive health services in Africa, Asia, and Latin America. Despite widespread agreement that the provision of health services of adequate quality is of fundamental importance to human welfare, the care available to women in the developing world is thought to be far from satisfactory. This suggests that in many cases providers have somehow failed to accomplish their goal to do good, although not always for reasons that are within their control.

In focusing here on health care for women we do not want to imply that the care provided to men is adequate, just that the accessibility and quality of services for women may be inferior (Das Gupta, 1989). The fact that life expectancy for males is actually lower than that for females in all but a few countries does not negate the importance of examining the health care available to women (Santow, 1994). Women enjoy a physiological advantage over men; therefore, making inferences about the quality of services for men and women from comparisons of age-specific mortality rates is potentially misleading.

The purpose of this chapter is to briefly review some of the issues related to quality of maternal and reproductive health services in developing countries that have emerged in the past few years, in particular those issues most salient to the midwifery profession. For this discussion, maternal and reproductive health services are broadly defined to include counselling, where relevant, and treatment or services for problems or concerns related to sexuality, physical abuse, reproductive-tract infections, other diseases of the reproductive organs, abortion, infertility, prenatal care, childbirth, and problems or concerns related to the menopause.

THE FOCUS ON TECHNICAL ASPECTS OF QUALITY

In the past, when quality of care was examined this was generally limited to an assessment of technical practices. This focus reflected the provider's concentration on the achievement of a narrow (albeit critical) set of health outcomes. For the staff working at the local health centre, reducing unwanted pregnancies, induced abortions, pregnancy and labour complications, and maternal and perinatal morbidity and mortality was of central importance. They were concerned with particular procedures or actions to be taken to achieve these outcomes. With regard to treatments and medications, providers want to avoid serious illness or death. Consequently, less attention is given to discomforts (usually not identified as illness), even if many patients are affected. To the extent, then, that quality of maternal health services was considered at all by the health establishment in developing countries, the focus was on those dimensions of care that are believed to reduce mortality and life-threatening morbidity.

An investigation of maternal deaths in Jamaica (Walker *et al.*, 1987) is but one example of a study in which inferences about quality were made from outcome data. Through hospital and coroner records, as well as death registration certificates, women who had died while pregnant or within a year of pregnancy were identified. Information was then gathered about each case and a summary assessment was developed and reviewed by obstetricians. Included in this assessment was a discussion of 'avoidable factors' that might have contributed to the death. This category included "the failure of the services to provide or offer adequate care," and was limited, quite justifiably given the outcome in question, to clinical procedures.

Yet there are many more examples of studies in which an evaluation of the interpersonal dimensions would seem an appropriate addition to the assessment of quality. For example, an examination of antenatal clinics in India (Srinivasa *et al.*, 1982), conducted nearly 20 years ago, used a check-list to assess history-taking, measurement of height and weight, recording of blood pressure, general physical and obstetric examination, haemoglobin estimation, urine analysis, tetanus toxoid administration, health education, explanation of prescription, and record maintenance. While this study was unusual in the depth of the information collected in the area of clinical competence, the more affective dimensions of quality were not considered at all. This same limitation characterizes an assessment of health facilities in rural Papua New Guinea (Garner *et al.*, 1990). In that study the focus was on the managerial determinants that affected the capacity of each health unit to perform specific tasks (e.g., immunization) or respond to particular situations (e.g., obstetric emergency and febrile convulsions in children).

INCORPORATING THE INTERPERSONAL DIMENSION

It has been the work of writers like Donabedian, alongside pressure from women's health advocates, that has widened the technical focus in the assessment of quality to include interpersonal dimensions. Although his own work was limited to health systems in the developed world, Donabedian made a seminal contribution to the debate in developing countries by emphasizing the interpersonal aspects of care, as well as such standard technical attributes as knowledge, judgement, and skill of the providers. The interpersonal domain consists of two-way patient–provider communication for the purpose of diagnosis, information exchange regarding the nature and management of the illness, and determination of the preference for treatment. Donabedian stressed that the relationship between patient and provider should be characterized by "privacy, confidentiality, informed choice, concern, empathy, honesty, tact, and sensitivity," arguing that the "interpersonal process is the vehicle by which technical care is implemented and on which its success depends" (Donabedian, 1988).

Feminists have also focused on an approach to health care that goes beyond clinical processes, arguing that a good-quality reproductive health service is one which promotes women's control over their own bodies, maintains health in its most comprehensive sense, and helps to improve sexual satisfaction.

These arguments, plus the widespread dissemination of the work of Donabedian, have resulted in an increasing interest in the assessment of services from the perspective of the individual client who receives care. Indeed, in the few documented situations in which the clients have been asked to define a high-quality health service, they generally provide a list of concrete attributes, many of which relate to the more interpersonal aspects of care. A study conducted at a family planning and maternal and infant care clinic in Santiago, Chile, which is probably generalizable to many patient populations, describes the concept of quality of care from the clients' viewpoint (Vera, 1993). For the women interviewed, quality of health services meant "being treated like a person, like a human being." Among the specific elements identified were (Vera, 1993):

- A clean, hygienic place.
- Prompt service.
- Accessible referral services.
- Useful and accurate information.
- Enough time to consult with staff about problems.
- Enough time to receive advice.
- An opportunity to learn.

- An opportunity to develop self-esteem.
- Treatment as an equal in transactions.
- Cordial, likeable, and friendly staff.
- Staff that are aware of the clients' learning needs.
- Access to the prescribed medications.
- An opportunity for husbands and partners to be educated.

Similarly, a study of clients' opinions of primary health care in Tanzania reported that (Gilson *et al.*, 1994):

> *Receiving the 'right' drugs from a rude health worker represented a poorer quality of care than receiving the same drugs from a polite worker, and perhaps was even poorer than receiving the 'wrong' drugs from a polite worker.*

QUALITY OF CARE – A FRAMEWORK FOR MATERNAL AND REPRODUCTIVE HEALTH SERVICES

The more holistic assessment of health services, labelled by Gilson *et al.* (1993) as 'process quality' and which includes interpersonal as well as technical skills, has rarely been undertaken in developing countries. In an effort to encourage a more systematic appraisal of the quality of care, and to expand the usual definition of quality beyond the technical aspects of care to incorporate the interpersonal dimensions mentioned by clients, Bruce (1990) developed a conceptual framework.

This framework, which defines quality of care for family planning and related reproductive services, has had a substantial impact on the international family planning community by providing a clear – and by now agreed upon – statement of what is meant by quality. The framework includes six elements: choice, technical information given to clients, technical competence, interpersonal relations, follow-up or continuity mechanisms, and an appropriate constellation of services.

Mensch (1992) has adapted the Bruce framework to the broader arena of women's health care. Although the elements remain the same, the indicators were modified. In developing a conceptual model for maternal and reproductive health services, we combine the elements of both frameworks and the indicators that Mensch listed. The following is a suggested list of elements and their corresponding indicators:

- *Choice* – Choice of treatment options and therapeutic regimes if medically appropriate and available.
- *Provider–client information exchange* – Conveying information to women, e.g. (a) explanation of the diagnosis; (b) information on treatment options; (c) information on the therapeutic regime; (d) information on contraindications to and side-effects of all medications and drugs; and (e) listening to and understanding women, including their background, preferences for treatment, and medical history.
- *Provider competence* – (a) accurate knowledge about the disease, problem, or condition; (b) technical proficiency in providing safe and appropriate clinical treatment known to produce an impact on mortality, morbidity, or the existing condition; and (c) knowledge of procedures for referring cases which cannot be managed adequately with the resources available.

- *Interpersonal relations* – sensitive treatment of women, including (a) privacy; (b) respectful and responsive provider behaviour; (c) encouragement of women's participation in decision making; (d) avoidance of moral judgement; (e) confidentiality; (f) limited waiting time; and (g) adequate amount of time spent with the woman.
- *Mechanisms to encourage continuity of medical care* – (a) information about when to return and, if possible, other locations where services and medications can be obtained; and (b) specific follow-up procedures including, when deemed necessary, future appointments and home visits.

This framework excluded the constellation or organizational structure of services because there is no *one* model or context for service delivery which is suitable in all settings (Kumar *et al.*, 1989). In the broad domain of women's health, it is not possible to state unequivocally what the best constellation of services is.

ASSESSING QUALITY IN MATERNAL AND REPRODUCTIVE HEALTH SERVICES

Many studies attribute maternal and reproductive morbidity and mortality to the inadequate quality of health services. (This is not to say that social and behavioural determinants of ill health are ignored in these studies, particularly when sexually transmitted diseases (STDs) are being considered.) Yet, as indicated earlier, systematic efforts to evaluate the quality of maternal health services have been lacking until very recently. This absence was partially due to the problems inherent in quantifying the elements of quality, although it was also due to the public health community's interest in promoting accessibility and availability of services without attention to the quality of these services. This interest reflected a belief that quality was a luxury that resource-constrained countries could ill-afford.

Responding to the growing interest in quality of care assessment, researchers have begun to develop tools to describe the services being provided. In the primary health-care field Gilson *et al.* (1993) have developed check-lists of "the series of expected actions required for the provision of good-quality care." The procedures included in the assessment are curative care for adults and children and specific nursing activities – injections, dispensing cleanliness, and sterilization. The check-lists were developed locally and are reflective of the accepted primary health-care practices in the region of Tanzania, where the assessment was undertaken. (Practices that resulted from resource constraints were not, however, 'condoned'.) Qualified medical assistants then used these check-lists to observe services in the dispensaries. The quality of antenatal services in this area was also evaluated through interviews with mothers, as well as through a comparison of patient records with independently obtained medical histories.

In the family planning field, the Population Council's Situation Analysis Methodology was developed partly to fulfil a programmatic need for information about the quality of services (Miller *et al.*, 1991; Fisher *et al.*, 1992). As is the case with the approach employed by Gilson (described above), this methodology uses observation rather than relying exclusively on interviews with staff and administrators. These studies typically include a large sample of service delivery points and attempt to produce a comprehensive appraisal of the service delivery point, including the major family planning subsystems (logistics, facilities, staffing, training, supervision, and record keeping), as well as the elements of quality (e.g., choice, provider–client information exchange, etc.).

Since 1989, the Population Council has undertaken situation analysis studies in 15 countries in Africa, Asia, and Latin America: Brazil, Burkina Faso, Côte d'Ivoire, Ghana, Guatemala, Kenya, Indonesia, Nigeria, Pakistan, Peru, Senegal, Tanzania, Turkey, Zaire, and Zimbabwe. Because the data generated by these assessments provide detailed information heretofore unavailable, the demand for such studies has grown rapidly. Indeed, many more surveys are underway or proposed. Interestingly, despite the variability in cultural settings and health infrastructures, there are some striking consistencies in the quality of family planning services across these countries. In general, provider–client information exchange is weak; family planning staff frequently do not discuss side-effects of methods with the clients and rarely inquire about any gynaecological problems the woman might have. Yet failure to provide adequate information may result in discontinuation of a contraceptive method should a problem develop. In addition, failure to investigate gynaecological problems may undermine reproductive health, especially if a contraindicated method is provided.

The situation analysis methodology has now been adapted to investigate the quality of other maternal health services, in addition to family planning. A module developed for pregnancy termination services is currently being tested in Turkey (AVSC/Turkey and Population Council, 1994). Using an assessment tool developed by the Population Council and the American College of Nurse-Midwives, the methodology is also being tested in Ghana and Vietnam to examine maternity care, including prenatal, labour, and delivery services. The study instruments for these countries contain sections on staffing, service statistics (patient information, treatment of complication, referrals), emergency transportation, status of referral sites, and clinical facilities (including infrastructure and storage of equipment and supplies). Of particular interest to midwives is a series of items that assess provider background and skills. Providers are also presented with hypothetical high-risk cases and are asked to delineate the appropriate management actions. Areas evaluated include the management of antenatal bleeding, puerperal sepsis, pre-eclampsia and eclampsia, postpartum haemorrhage, and protracted labour (Sloan et al., 1994).

The purpose of these assessments is to determine the requirements for upgrading facilities and training so that adequate emergency obstetric services can be provided in the health communes, field hospitals, and district hospitals.

The preliminary data from both Ghana and Vietnam reveal similar weaknesses in service delivery. At the commune or health-post level, midwife training, facility upgrading, and improved transportation systems are clearly needed. In particular, midwife knowledge of how to manage obstetric emergencies is generally poor, especially with regard to antenatal bleeding, sepsis, pre-eclampsia and eclampsia, and retained placenta. The goal is to use these data as a baseline from which the process of improving the quality of maternity care in Ghana and Vietnam can begin (Taylor et al., 1994 and Hieu et al., 1994, respectively).

STRATEGIES FOR IMPROVING THE QUALITY OF CARE IN MATERNAL AND REPRODUCTIVE HEALTH SERVICES

If the quality of maternal health care in developing countries is to improve, it is essential that policymakers and donor agencies make this an explicit item on their agendas. Without this commitment, it is difficult to envision how services can change for the better.

In an attempt to upgrade services for women, it is important to describe the *four steps* involved in the care-giving improvement process (Jain *et al.*, 1992). The process should be clear-cut and should be made operational through on-going dialogues that include both managers and providers, and afford a voice for clients. It should seek to answer the following questions (Jain *et al.*, 1992):

- What quality of care does the health system intend to offer?
- What quality of care is it prepared to offer?
- What quality of care is actually offered?
- What quality of care is received by the clients?

The *first step* is to articulate the minimum standards that are acceptable and affordable. The managers and providers should be clear about the norms and standards of care they wish to offer their clients. The standards should include all elements of care, interpersonal and informational, as well as clinical. Then a set of explicit statements concerning the standard should be prepared.

The *second step* calls for programme managers' judgement about whether the infrastructure is adequate to offer the care that policy dictates. Damiba (1992), in his work with family planning programmes in West Africa, describes this process with the assistance of a visual aid (see *Figure 13.1*):

> *Quality of care can be viewed as a pyramid with the base corresponding to the service delivery infrastructure, the middle level consisting of program management, and the crown of the pyramid being the services offered.*

Figure 13.1 emphasizes the importance of addressing quality-of-care issues from the ground level. Improving the quality of the work place through infrastructure

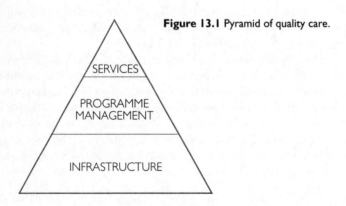

Figure 13.1 Pyramid of quality care.

renovations (equipment and facilities, staff training and supervision, record keeping and supplies) is a needed, but not sufficient, prerequisite for improving the quality of services offered to women.

The *third step* asks if the staff are offering the services as planned. The *fourth step* views the care giving process from the clients' perspective. These two steps can be assessed by observing the client–provider transactions and interviewing women, as is done in the situation analysis and Gilson studies described earlier. Although observation of care is sometimes perceived as technically difficult, inconvenient, and intrusive, it apparently provides more objective data than do staff interviews. The client's perspective can be best understood by observing a sample of women from beginning to end of the service transaction, as well as interviewing these women.

A description of the standards of quality that are desired, as well as of the care offered and received, is crucial. However, it is also important to develop a managerial agenda to improve the quality of reproductive health services. Huntington *et al.* (1993) have developed such an agenda consisting of four elements:

- Enhance the autonomy of service providers, in terms of the material resources available and the training provided for their work.
- Develop a strategy for quality assurance that focuses on a continual process of participatory supervision, in-service training, and personal investment from front-line workers to provide quality services.
- Develop a programmatic focus on improving the working conditions of front-line workers and mid-level managers, rather than simply expanding the current status to new sites.
- Develop a wider base of support for health services by building the participation of community leaders into the quality assurance programme.

QUALITY OF CARE – CHALLENGES FOR THE FUTURE AND THE ROLE OF MIDWIVES

The quality-of-care framework discussed here is a starting point meant to provoke debate among those who provide maternal and reproductive health services in developing countries. It is not meant to be used as a rigid tool, but as a practical and analytical one. The challenges that lie ahead may differ for each health service. Each programme may choose to give different emphasis to different elements of quality, depending on the maturity of the health system and the political and economic constraints it faces.

This discussion should lead to a more comprehensive understanding of the various dimensions involved in improving the quality of maternal and reproductive health services, and simultaneously draw attention to the programme–client interface as a critical and neglected dimension in programme effort. It is important to emphasize that the recommendations for future action, both in policy and research, focus not just on the technical aspects of quality, but also on the interpersonal dimensions.

Simmons and Elias (1994) have further defined this interpersonal dimension – the client–provider interaction – in terms of both its manifest and latent dimensions. Manifest dimensions include the quality-of-care elements defined by Bruce (1990), the frequency and duration of the interactions, and other variables which can influence the nature of the services provided [types of contraceptive methods provided, other reproductive health services offered (e.g., STD counselling and treatment), and non-professional functions performed (conflict mediation and financial counselling)].

The latent dimension, while relatively hidden, is nonetheless a critical feature of the client–provider interaction. It involves 'status, power, and the culture' of the participants in the encounter. These are especially important in traditional societies (Simmons and Elias, 1994):

> *where clients often experience providers as powerful individuals, whose social background and training are far removed from clients' daily realities and concerns.*

It is on the interpersonal aspect of quality of care, in particular the latent dimension, that midwives will have the greatest impact. Midwives have viewed their role in the broadest sense, not only as purveyors of the technologies, but as sources of continuing support for clients as their needs change. Moreover, midwifery has a philosophical commitment to choice in all aspects of maternal health services. As providers in community-based programmes, midwives are in a key position to listen to the voices of those who work on the front line: the field-worker and other services providers (outreach worker, volunteers, medical–paramedical personnel) at the clinic and community level.

Strict hierarchical management styles, and cultural and community norms, can often have a negative influence on the behaviour of health care personnel. Supportive communication will be inhibited, a trusting relationship between client and provider will not develop, and many individuals will avoid contact with maternal health service programmes. To prevent this eventuality, midwives need to provide impetus for a 'reorientation' process. This process involves a willingness on the part of providers to reorient their work towards consideration of the latent dimensions of the client–provider interaction. It involves increasing sensitivity to the needs of clients and to the personal, social, and cultural factors involved in reproductive health. Midwives can conduct workshops with staff to elicit their attitudes towards clients, and brainstorm regarding strategies for handling various problems. A possible approach would be to engage providers in a review of hypothetical situations. In this way, some of the constraints that providers experience can be revealed in a non-threatening manner. Once an understanding exists of how clients and providers interact, midwives can begin to see how operational, managerial, structural, or policy variables support or hinder productive relationships; they can then foster change at these points in the service delivery system.

Midwifery can serve as a bridge between front-line workers, managers, and policymakers. It can assist in the development and initiation of changes required to bring service delivery standards to their intended level.

The next decade will be a challenging time for those concerned with reducing reproductive morbidity, maternal mortality, unsafe abortion, and unwanted child-bearing in the developing world. Explicit attention to quality of services will help providers determine which aspects of care have the greatest impact on these health outcomes. In that midwifery by its very nature is client-oriented, midwives should feature prominently in these efforts to improve the quality of maternal and reproductive health services.

ACKNOWLEDGEMENTS

This chapter has drawn heavily on the following: Kumar *et al.*, 1989; Bruce, 1990; Bruce and Jain, 1991; Jain *et al.*, 1992; Mensch, 1992; Huntington *et al.*, 1993; and Simmons and Elias, 1994.

REFERENCES

AVSC/Turkey and Population Council (1994) *Situation Analysis of Turkey's Family Planning and Pregnancy Termination Services*. Proposal submitted to the United States Agency for International Development.

Bruce, J. (1990) Fundamental elements of the quality of care: a simple framework. *Studies in Family Planning*, **21**(2): 61–91.

Bruce, J. and Jain, A.K. (1991) Improving quality of care through operations research. In: Seidman, M. and Horn, M. (eds), *Operations Research: Helping Family Planning Programs Work Better*. John Wiley & Sons, New York.

Damiba, A. (1992) *SEATS: Experience for Improving Family Planning Services*. Unpublished paper presented at the Francophone Quality of Care Conference, Senegal, 6–7 February (cited in Huntington *et al.*, 1993).

Das Gupta, M. (1989) Effects of discrimination on health and mortality. In: *Proceedings of the International Population Conference*, New Dehli, Vol. 3, pp 349–365. International Union for the Scientific Study of Population, Liege, Belgium,.

Donabedian, A. (1988) The quality of care: how can it be assessed? *Journal of the American Medical Association*, **260**(12): 1743–1748.

Faundes, A. (1990) *Quality of Care in Postpartum Contraception*. Paper presented at the International Conference on Postpartum Contraception, Mexico City. Unpublished.

Fisher, A., Mensch, B.S., Miller, R.A., Askew, I., Jain, A.K., Ndeti, C., Ndhlovu, L., and Tapsoba, P. (1992) *Guidelines and Instruments for a Family Planning Situation Analysis Study*. The Population Council, New York.

Garner, P., Thomason, J., and Donaldson, D. (1990) Quality assessment of health facilities in rural Papua New Guinea. *Health Policy and Planning*, **5**(1): 49–59.

Gilson, L., Kitange, H., and Teuscher, T. (1993) Assessment of process quality in Tanzanian primary care. *Health Policy*, **26**: 119–139.

Gilson, L., Alilio, M., and Heggenhougen, K. (1994) Community satisfaction with primary health care services: an evaluation undertaken in the Morogoro region of Tanzania. *Social Science and Medicine*, **39**(6): 767–780.

Hieu, Do Trong, Ngoc, Nguyen Thi, Nhu, Hau, Nguyen Trong, Sloan, N., Quimby, C., Schwalbe, N., and Winikoff, B. (1994) *Selected Findings from a Situation Analysis of Emergency Obstetric Services in Two Provinces in Vietnam*. Appendix to an interim progress report for the Safe Motherhood Demonstration Project submitted to the World Bank, Washington, DC, by the Population Council, New York.

Huntington, D., Thome, M., and Seck, M. (1993) *Report from the Francophone Africa Quality of Care Conference*. Population Council Regional Working Paper Series, No. 2. The Population Council, Dakar, Senegal.

Jain, A.K., Bruce, J., and Mensch, B.S. (1992) Setting standards of quality in family planning programs. *Studies in Family Planning*, **23**(6): 392–395.

Kumar, S., Jain, A.K., and Bruce, J. (1989) *Assessing the Quality of Family Planning Services in Developing Countries*. Programs Division Working Paper Series, No. 2. The Population Council, New York.

Mensch, B.S. (1992) Quality of care: a neglected dimension. In: Koblinsky, M.A., Timyan, J., and Gay, J. (eds), *The Health of Women: A Global Perspective*, Boulder. Westview Press, Colorado.

Miller, R.A., Ndhlovu, L., and Gachara, M.M. (1991) The situation analysis study of the family planning program in Kenya. *Studies in Family Planning*, **22**(3): 131–143.

Roemer, M.I. and Montoya-Aguilar, C. (1988) *Quality Assessment and Assurance in Primary Health Care*. World Health Organization, Geneva.

Santow, G. (1994) Book review of 'The health of women: a global perspective'. *Health Transition Review*, **4**(2): 245–246.

Simmons, R. and Elias, C. (1994) The study of client–provider interactions: a review of methodological issues. *Studies in Family Planning*, **25**(1): 1–17.

Sloan, N., Quimby, C., Winikoff, B., and Schwalbe, N. (1994) *Guidelines and Instruments for a Maternity Care Situation Analysis Study*. Appendix to the interim progress report for the Safe Motherhood Demonstration Project submitted to the World Bank, Washington, DC, by the Population Council, New York.

Srinivasa, D.K., Danabalan, M., and Rangachari, R. (1982) Method to assess quality of services in antenatal clinics of primary health centres. *Indian Journal of Medical Research*, **76**: 458–466.

Subcommittee on Quality Indicators in Family Planning Service Development (1990) *Report of the Subcommittee on Quality Indicators in Family Planning Services*, Washington, J. Helzner (Chair). Unpublished paper submitted to the Task Force on Standardization of Family Planning Performance Indicators, New York.

Taylor, J., Sakyi-Ajei, K., Arthur, P., Paxton, A., and Sloan, N. (1994) *Preliminary Draft: Ghana Situation Analysis*. Appendix to the interim progress report of the Safe Motherhood Demonstration Project submitted to the World Bank, New York, Population Council, New York.

United Nations (1991) *The World's Women 1970–1990: Trends and Statistics*. Social Statistics and Indicators Series K, No. 8. United Nations Department of Discrimination on Health and Social Affairs, New York.

Vera, H. (1993) The client's view of high quality care in Santiago, Chile. *Studies in Family Planning*, **24**(1): 40–49.

Walker, G.J.A., Ashley, D.E.C., McCaw, A.M., and Bernard, G.W. (1987) Maternal deaths in Jamaica. *World Health Forum*, **8**: 75–79.

Index